ultimate**makeovers**

ultimate**makeovers**

expert makeup secrets for
stunning transformations including
weddings and special occasions

by robert jones

beauty
robert jones

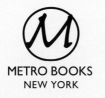

METRO BOOKS
NEW YORK

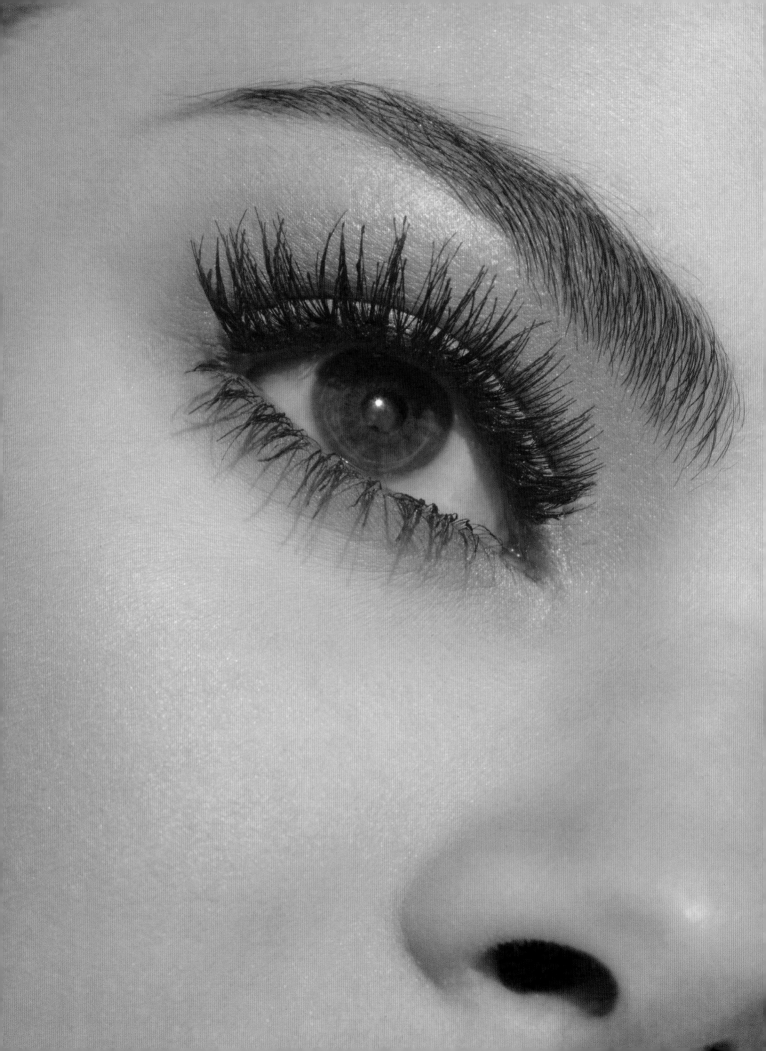

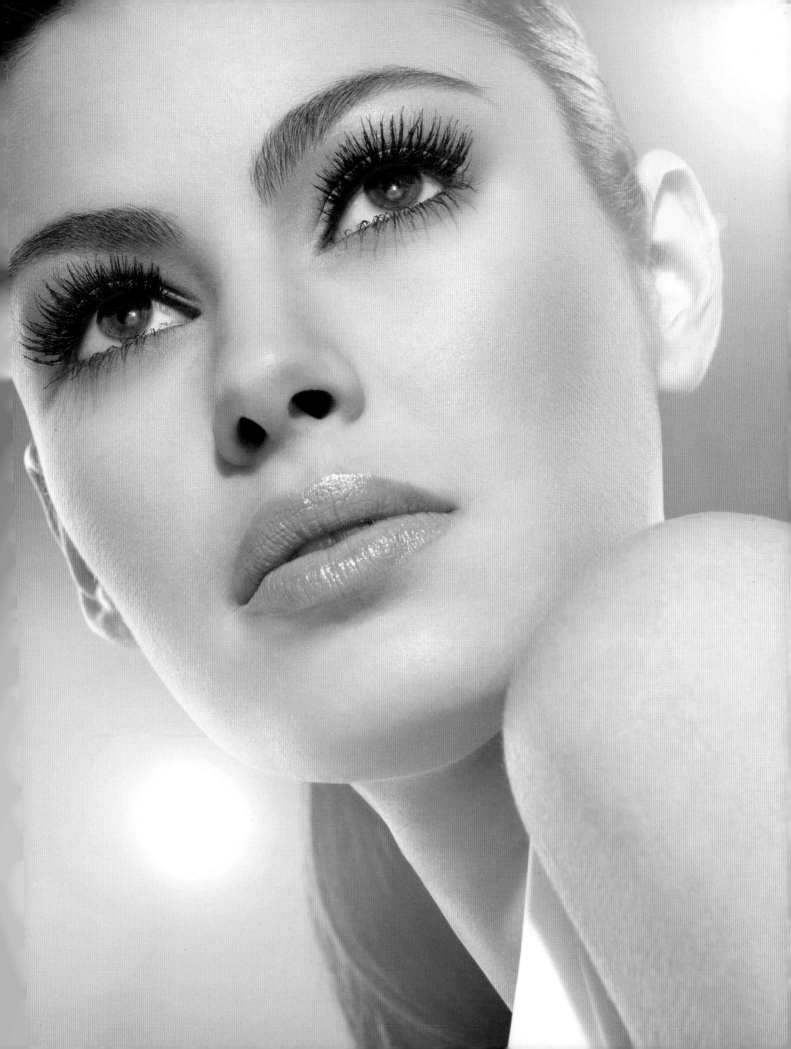

This 2008 edition published by Metro Books by arrangement with
Fair Winds Press, a member of Quayside Publishing Group.

Quayside Publishing Group
100 Cummings Center
Suite 406-L
Beverly, MA 01915-6101
www.quaysidepublishinggroup.com

Text by Robert Jones and Lisa Bower
Hair and makeup by Robert Jones, assisted by Susie Jasper, Missy Brumley,
and Lisa Williams
Representation by Seaminx Artist Management, www.seaminx.com
Produced by Elaine Moock, Sunni Smyth, and Tiffany Mullen
Fashion and beauty photography by Jeff Stephens
Fashion styling by Chad Curry
Still-life photography by Fernando Ceja
Still-life styling by Phillip Groves
Illustrations by Robin Kachantones
Jewelry courtesy of H2 herrenhuffaker, www.herrenhuffaker.com
Flowers courtesy of M. Bountiful, a flower shop in Dallas
Bridal gowns courtesy of Saks Fifth Avenue, Galleria Dallas, Stanley Korshak Dallas,
Neiman Marcus Downtown Dallas, and Myrdith Leon-McCormack New York
Special thanks to Patty Woodrich for her never-ending support (I could not have
done this without her) and Michael Glassmoyer for his original vision!
robertjonesbeauty.com

Metro Books
122 Fifth Avenue
New York, NY 10011

ISBN-13: 978-1-4351-0911-7

Printed and bound in China

1 3 5 7 9 10 8 6 4 2

This book is dedicated to four very special people. Three have passed through my life, each of whom I believe are now watching from above as guardian angels: my grandmother, Carolyn Walker Scoville, who inspired me to love beauty; Bernardo Aldrete, no one ever believed in me more; and Diane Payne, a true inspiration. Finally, the most important, and here with me: Chip McFadin, the love of my life, my rock.

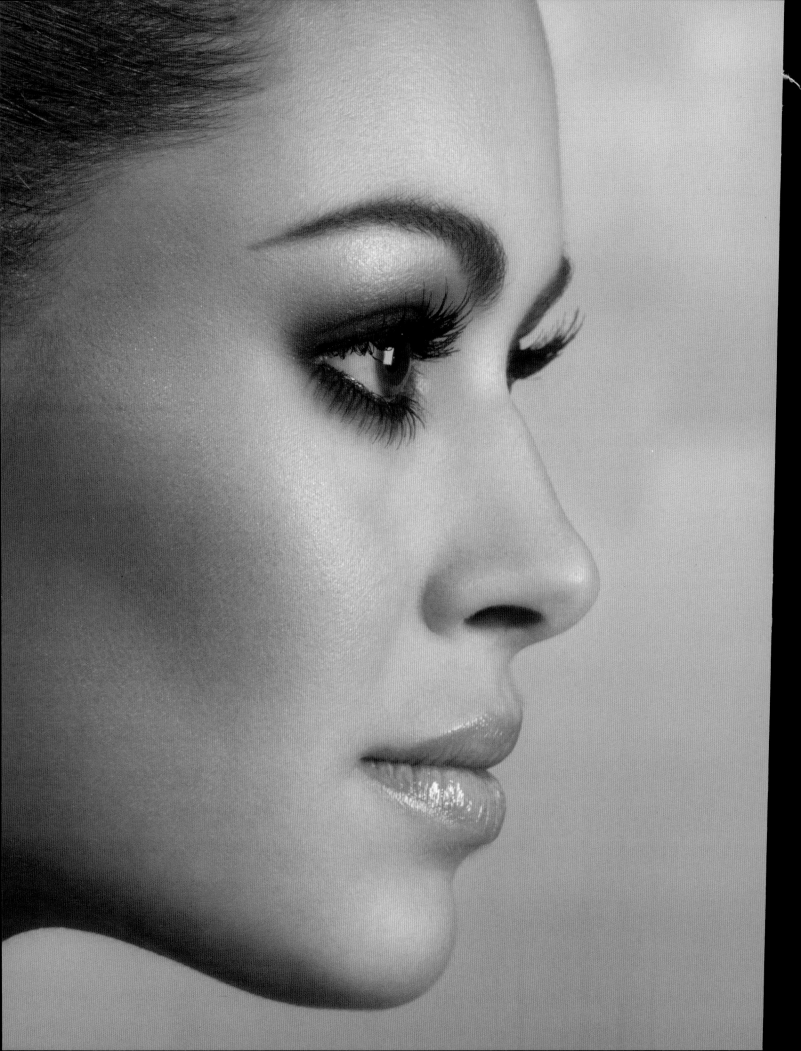

embrace your own personal beauty—love who you are today and everyday.

—robert jones

part one getting ready

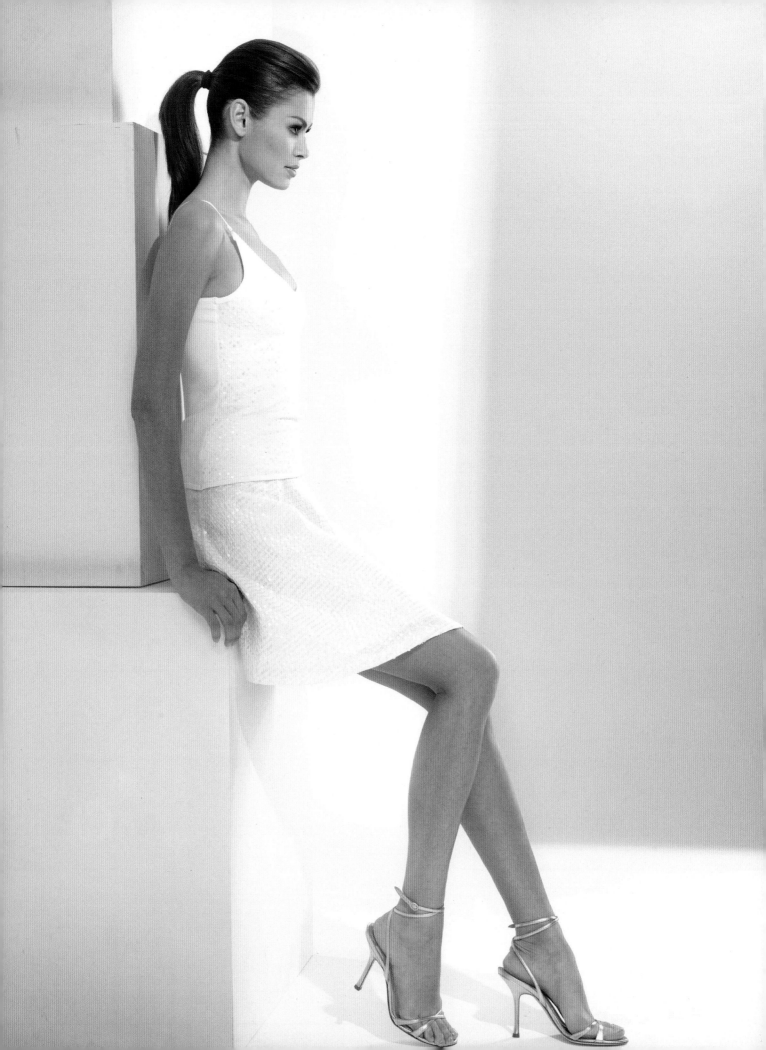

truebeauty

This book is all about you—who you are, who you want to be, and who you can be. I truly feel that every woman is beautiful. It is just a matter of recognizing your beauty and making it your focus.

I have long been convinced that beauty is not just about possessing a perfectly symmetrical face. Obviously, it's marvelous to be blessed with exceptional features, but not all of the women I've made up in my many years as a professional makeup artist were flawless. Some of the most beautiful women I have ever seen or worked with are beautiful because of who they are and what comes from within. Beauty comes from the expression and character in your face—not just its symmetry. It doesn't matter if you are short or tall, heavy or thin, or if your features aren't those of a fashion model or famous actress. Your beauty comes from self-awareness, self-confidence, and your own magnetic personality. Actually, I feel that self-confidence is the most important element of true beauty.

My goal in writing this book is to help you bring out that beauty from within by increasing your self-confidence about your outward appearance. I want to demystify the art of makeup and help you understand how to use it as a tool to better appreciate who you are. Some women think makeup is far too difficult to master, but it's simple when you break it down. It's merely a matter of using the right products, good tools, and the correct techniques.

First and most importantly, let me say that every woman needs to remember she is beautiful. By identifying your most striking features and accentuating them, we can make you look and feel more beautiful. Certainly one of the reasons I love being a makeup artist is the joy it gives me when I see how my work can change the way you feel about yourself. No matter what your age, if you are beautifully made up with bright eyes and a healthy glow, you will exude an aura of confidence that will draw people to you.

LESS IS MORE

Modern makeup should be simple and natural so it's the face we notice—not the makeup. I feel that cosmetics are to enhance the features God gave you, not to change them. I'm not suggesting natural makeup means walking around all day looking washed out. By simple and natural, I mean your makeup palette should be suited to your complexion and should change with each season to complement the change in your skin's natural tone. Sometimes I'll notice a woman who obviously has made an effort with her makeup but has chosen a foundation color that's all wrong for her skin tone, or she's wearing a lip color that's far too dark or vivid for her. The concept that "less is more" definitely holds true for makeup.

Makeup is meant to be beautiful, and beautiful makeup is all about the colors you choose and where you place them—never about how much you put on. I also think that it is important to remember that the face is not flat. It's not one-dimensional, therefore don't paint it that way. Makeup should be used to artfully sculpt and accentuate your best features—that is the very essence and purpose of wearing makeup.

YOUR MAKEUP MAKEOVER

Keep in mind that there are very few hard-and-fast rules in makeup and beauty. Beauty is in the eye of the beholder. And since beauty is subjective, everything discussed in this book reflects my own personal views. Each professional makeup artist has his or her own style, as do each of you. Mine has been described by many as the 'Glamorous-Girl-Next-Door'—I guess because I think all women should look beautiful but be approachable, and a little glamour never hurts. I want to help you discover your own personal style. Whatever the season or event, beautiful makeup will boost your self-confidence, which in turn will make you feel good about yourself, which will translate into true beauty. So read on—experiment with your makeup— have fun with it, and together we'll discover a more self-confident and beautiful you.

Makeup is meant to be beautiful, and beautiful makeup is all about the colors you choose and where you place them—never about how much you put on.

—robert jones

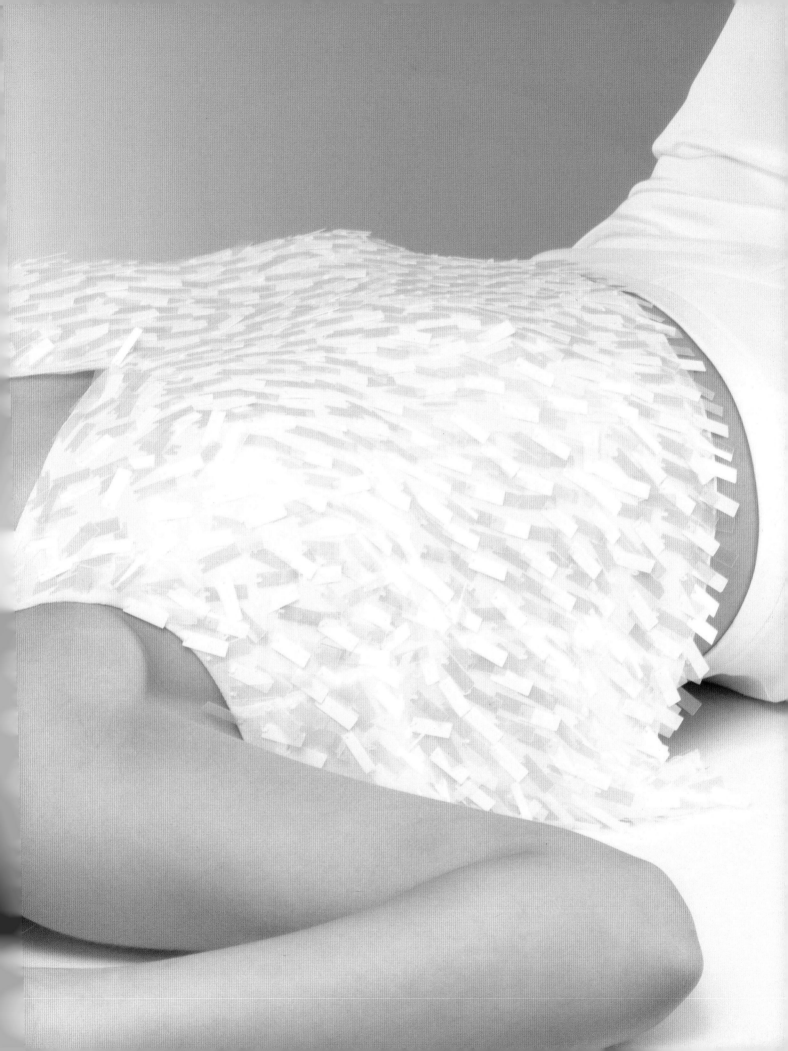

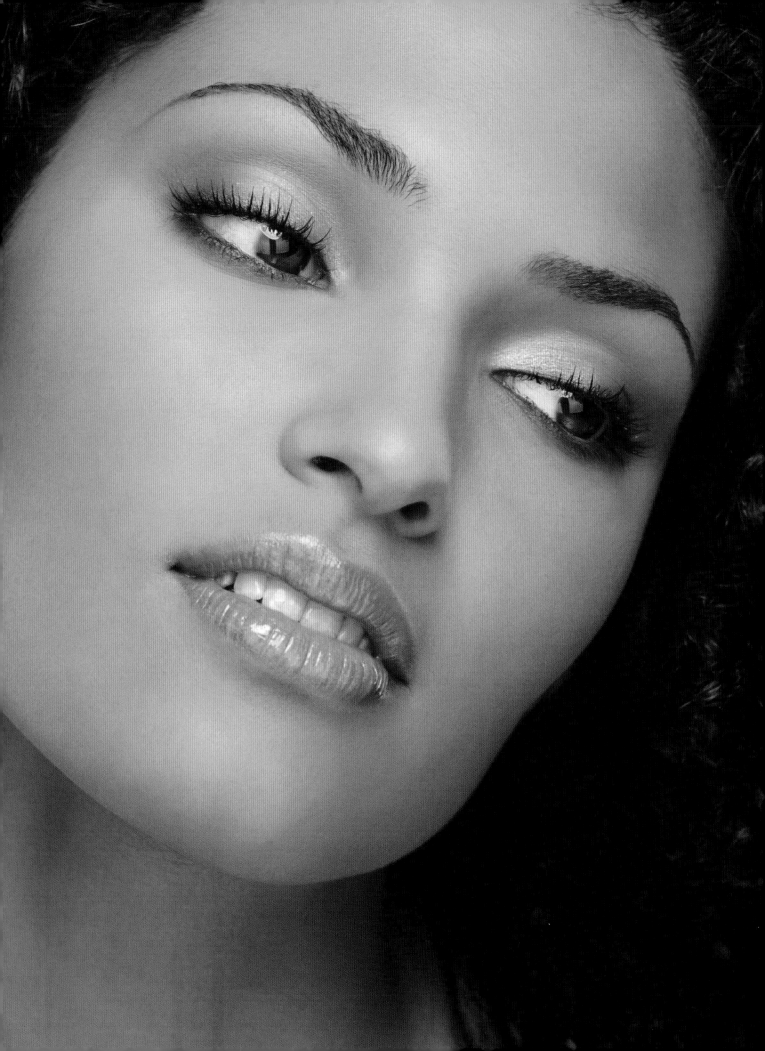

thewords

Mastering the art of makeup application begins with knowing some of the basic terms. As you read through the next couple of pages, you'll find the definitions for some of the most commonly used words in the makeup business. Get to know and understand them, and you'll soon be talking like a makeup pro.

Blush is for adding a wonderfully warm glow to the face. It can brighten the dullest of skin. If your cheeks are naturally rosy you might skip the blush and leave the glow up to Mother Nature.

Concealer is a miracle product that hides everything your foundation doesn't. It makes broken capillaries, undereye circles, age spots and any skin discolorations disappear.

Contour is the opposite of highlight. Everything that we contour we push away from the eye to make it appear less visible. A "contour" shade is usually a darker shade that gives your features more depth and definition by contrasting against the lighter shades used on your face and around the eyes. Contouring is also the last step in the three-color layering technique for the eyes.

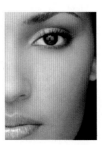

Dewy often refers to foundation finishes that create a fresh and glowing look with a slight sheen.

Eyeliner is for defining and "bringing out" the eyes, though it is not always necessary.

Eyeshadow is either applied lightly as a gentle color wash or as a more dramatic layering of color and texture to enhance and add shape to the eyes.

Foundation is a miracle product that evens out your complexion and covers imperfections. Your foundation's tone depends entirely on your skin. If your skin is looking radiant and beautiful without help, then by all means skip the foundation and go to a light dusting of powder. However, if you do need foundation, it comes in a variety of texture finishes such as matte, satin, and dewy. If you have oily or blemished skin, choose matte. If your skin is normal or dry, you can choose from any of the finishes.

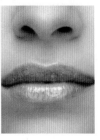

Frost is about maximum sparkle and super-shine. It is also sometimes referred to as iridescent. It is a fun, sexy look and works best on young skin because on more mature skin, it can draw attention to the fine lines. The term is usually used in reference to eyeshadows and lip color.

Gloss is a super high-shine lip color. It can add a punch of color, but does not stay on as long as lipstick.

Highlight is the opposite of contour. Everything you highlight comes toward you and helps draw attention to a specific area or feature. A highlight shade is usually a lighter shade used on the face and the eyes. Highlighting is the first step in the three-color layering technique for the eyes.

Lip color is the quickest way to set the mood of your overall look. You can go all out and define your lips with color, or you can smear a clear gloss or healing lip balm for that pared-down, natural look.

Luminescence describes a foundation with light-reflecting qualities that creates a glowing, refined look. The light-reflecting properties contain specially shaped particles that bounce light away from surface lines and wrinkles to create a more youthful look.

Mascara gives you those full, long, thick, and dark lashes you've always wanted. If I've just described your natural lashes, an eyelash curler may be all it takes to spotlight your baby blues, browns, grays, or greens. (If marooned on a desert island, mascara would be the number one makeup product most women would like to have with them.)

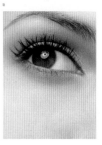

Matte is used to describe lipsticks, eyeshadows, foundations, powders, and blushes that have absolutely no shine and appear flat. Matte lipsticks tend to be drier, but they stay on much longer. Matte foundations are excellent on shiny and oily skins and are best for imperfect complexions. There are also matte products such as powders and crèmes that will help fight oils during the day.

Metallic describes lipsticks, eye-shadows, and eye pencils that have a shiny, metal finish. It's a look that's fantastic on ebony or darker skin, but too harsh for lighter or more mature skin.

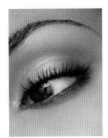

Midtone is a neutral, natural eye color that you sweep across the eyelids to help define and shape the eyes. The midtone shade should be a natural extension of your complexion and is the second step in the three-color layering technique for the eyes.

Opaque is a finish that provides absolute coverage, allowing nothing to show through.

Porosity is the skin's ability to hold moisture. Moisturizer can "even out" the porosity of your skin and help your foundation, primer, or concealer go on more smoothly.

Powder is for setting foundation. It gives your face a smooth finish and keeps shine under control.

Satin refers to a formulation that's neither as flat as matte nor as shiny as shimmer. A "soft satin finish" is often used to describe foundations and liquid cosmetics that give a soft, smooth finish to the skin. Satin products have a sheen to them but are not shiny. Satin eyeshadows are particularly good for mature skin because they glide on smoothly and add a soft sheen to the skin.

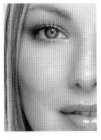

Sheer is a thinner and more transparent finish that gives the skin a glow. It usually contains silicone that allows makeup to glide on easily. The product clings less and covers more smoothly without being opaque. Sheer products seem to disappear into the skin, giving it a soft, more natural appearance. Sheer foundation is fabulous for mature women since it helps their skin appear brighter and fresher without drawing attention to fine lines. And it's perfect for younger skin tones that need to be evened out.

Stippling is a blending technique used for concealers and foundations. It's especially effective for blending out the edges of concealers. It is a patting motion, usually done with your fingers or a sponge. Stippling is also a great way to carefully apply one product over another. Just place some product, such as foundation, on your fingertips or a sponge and apply in a gentle patting motion so as not to disturb or erase the product you've already applied underneath, such as concealer.

Texture is the finish a product gives you—the way it appears on your skin. For example, a blush can have a creamy or a powdery texture. Foundation can have a dewy, creamy, sheer, matte, or satin texture. Lipsticks can be glossy, matte, or sheer. It's always wise to match your textures powder on powder, crème on crème.

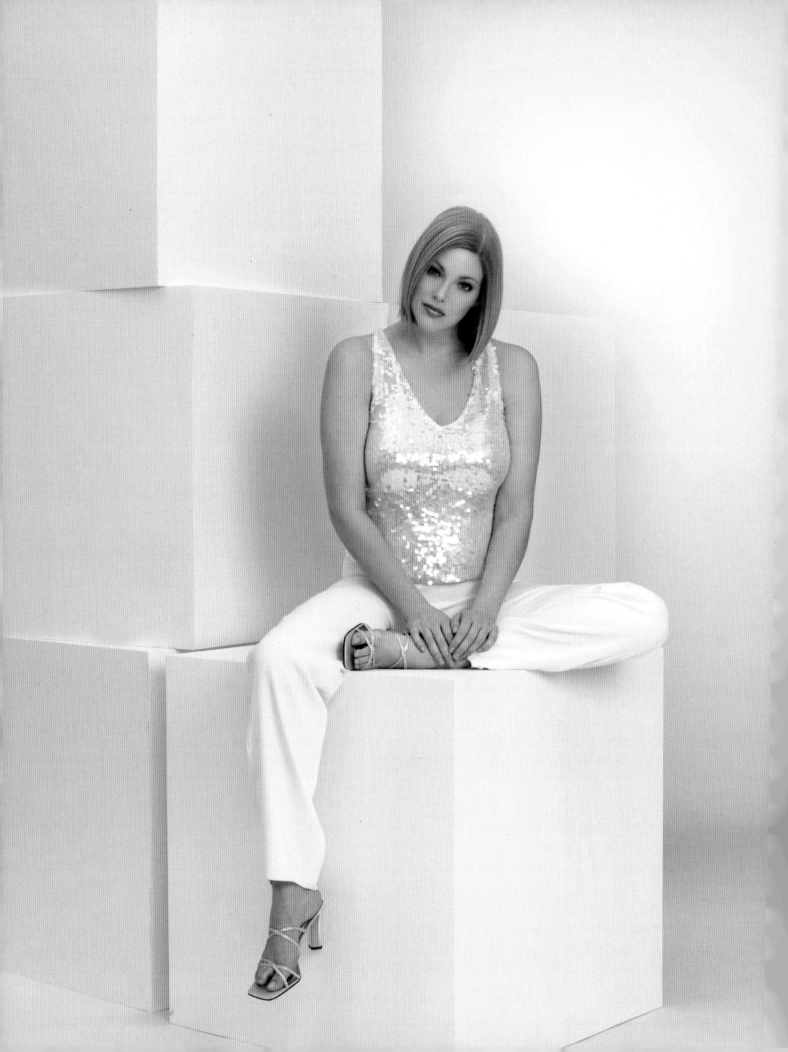

product**knowledge**

3

With so many products out there, it sometimes seems hard to know which one is right for you. Well, never fear. Together, we'll talk about the various makeup products, their forms and what makes them unique, and how to use each one. Aren't you feeling more confident already?

foundation

is your most important makeup investment. It can make your skin appear flawless and natural, and give it a healthy glow. It can cover imperfections and blemishes, and smooth out uneven skin tones. Wearing it correctly can do more for your appearance than practically any other makeup product. It can also be one of the most difficult to choose correctly.

When making your foundation choice, there are two things to consider. The first is to match your skin tone and depth so that your foundation looks natural. Secondly, it's important to match your skin type with the correct foundation formula. For example, if you have oily skin, sometimes the oils from your skin can mix with the product and make your foundation appear blotchy and uneven. Wearing the correct foundation formula for your skin type can help your foundation stay on longer.

My advice? Spend generously on your foundation. The difference in cost of cosmetics from one company to another is not only because of the packaging, but also because of the ingredients. The purer the ingredients, the more expensive a product will be. Higher-priced foundations usually contain a higher quality of pigments, which last longer on your skin and appear much more flattering. Cheaper foundations contain fewer and inferior pigments that usually don't wear as long. If you want to treat yourself, splurge on the best foundation you can afford to buy. Foundation and powder are the bases of your look, and therefore the most important makeup products. Save your pennies on less expensive color products so you can afford to play around and have fun with color.

Thanks to modern technology, we have many advanced foundations to work with, and they can appear almost invisible. You can choose from a variety of textures and formulas that will give you different types of coverage and finishes. A product's consistency and the way it actually goes onto the skin is the key to even, flawless coverage. The real goal for your foundation is for it to look as if you're not wearing any at all. You simply give the illusion of having healthy, beautiful skin.

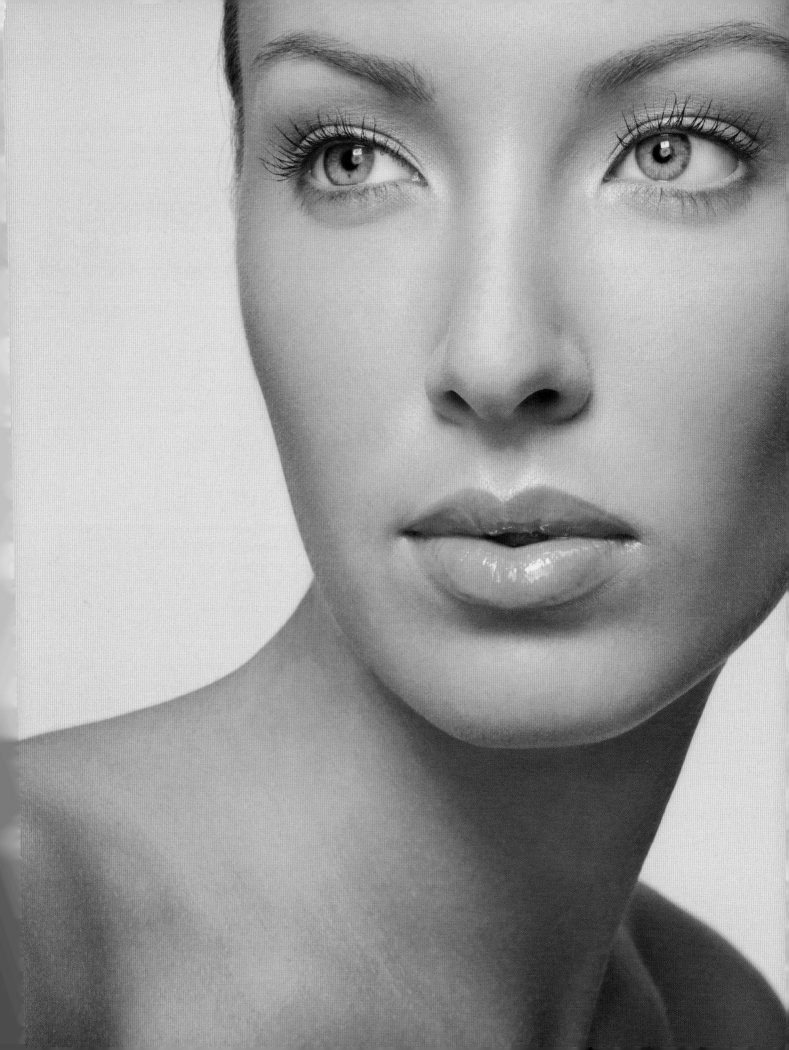

FOUNDATION GENERALLY COMES IN EIGHT DIFFERENT FORMS:

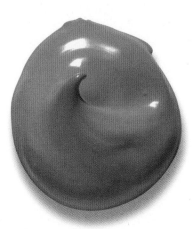

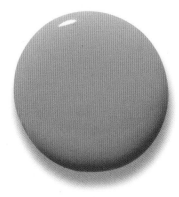

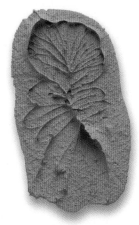

Stick foundation is essentially a neatly packaged crème foundation and concealer in one. Best for normal to dry skin, it is a good option for women who want more coverage. It offers ideal maximum coverage for imperfections as well as covering ruddy and uneven skin tones. Stick foundation will give you quick coverage, but it can look a little heavy on clear skin where a lot of coverage is not needed.

Liquid foundation is the most readily found and is suited to most—if not all—skin types. It is available in formulations from oil-free, oil-absorbing formulas to moisturizing formulas and gives varying degrees of sheer to medium coverage depending on the brand and the formula. You can purchase liquid foundation in a bottle or a tube. When applied, it gives you more coverage than a tinted moisturizer but less than a crème foundation.

Crème foundation is smooth and creamy and is specifically formulated for dry-to-normal complexions. It gives the skin a natural finish while offering the highest coverage. I find it to be the most versatile, because even though it tends to be of a thicker and heavier consistency, it can be made sheerer simply by applying it with a damp sponge. Also, because of its great coverage, it can even be used as a concealer if you don't have severe under-eye circles. Crème foundation is great for dry skin; however, if you have dry, flaky skin, beware, because it can look "cakey" and the result can be slightly dull and heavy-looking.

Mousse foundation is actually a crème foundation that has a whipped consistency. It generally comes in a jar rather than a compact, and it is usually lighter and sheerer than its compact counterpart. It evens out the skin tone without appearing heavy. I use mousse-textured formulas a lot because they seem to sink into the skin rather than sit on top of it. They give great coverage that appears very natural. They are fabulous on mature skin because they do not collect in fine lines like heavier crème formulas.

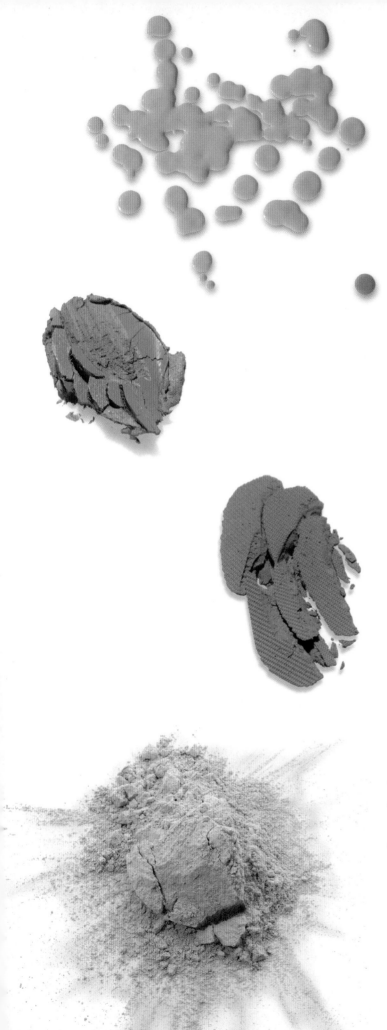

Tinted moisturizer is actually a moisturizer with a little color added. It's the sheerest of all the foundations, and it's perfect for use during the summer months when you feel like wearing next to nothing. It evens out the skin tone while providing minimal coverage.

Crème-to-powder foundation is quick and simple. It has a creamy texture that dries to a powder finish, so usually no additional dusting of powder is needed to set it. These formulas are kinder to oily skin than their crème counterparts because the powder helps cut down on excess shine.

Powder compact is a dual-finish powder foundation that gives a quick and convenient sheer to medium coverage. It is simply a pressed powder that can be used wet or dry. Used dry, it goes on like a pressed powder but gives you slightly more coverage. I find that it's perfect for young girls because it's low in oils and doesn't clog pores, and so there's little risk of pimples appearing without warning. And it's great for touch-ups when you're on the go. Applied with a brush, it gives you sheer coverage. Applied with a sponge, it gives you more coverage. Applied with a damp sponge, it gives you even more complete coverage, more like liquid and crème foundations.

Pigmented mineral powder is simply a loose powder that adheres to the skin, providing medium to full coverage. In addition to giving you coverage it also contains vitamins and minerals to help treat the skin. It works much like a dual-finish powder foundation and is simple to apply with a brush or a sponge.

concealer

comes in various formulations and textures. Different textures of concealers are used on different problem areas, so it's important to match the texture with the problem area. For example, a concealer used to cover under-eye areas should always be moist and creamy, whereas a concealer designed to cover breakouts or broken capillaries should be much drier in texture so it will adhere better and last longer.

Solid cream stick concealers give full coverage but are not always the easiest to blend. They are used primarily for hiding some of the more prominent blemishes and skin discoloration. They can also be used to minimize under-eye circles, but if you're going to use this texture, make sure the consistency is creamy enough to blend well so as not to accentuate fine lines. Since the most delicate skin is under the eyes, using a hard-to-blend stick concealer can actually make the circles look far worse by drawing attention to them.

Pot concealer provides similar coverage to stick, but it is usually formulated with more moisturizing ingredients and is not quite as thick—much better for underneath the eyes. This is the concealer that's probably the most commonly used by professionals because of the great coverage it gives. Although usually creamy, it is also available in drier, oil-free formulas that are used to cover discoloration on the rest of the face.

Tube concealer has a creamier texture that is lighter and less likely to collect in fine lines, making it great for mature skin. It's also one of the most versatile forms of concealer. It provides terrific coverage and can be mixed with moisturizer or foundation to create a much sheerer product. It's also perfect to use under the eyes because it's one of the easiest to blend.

Wand concealers offer the lightest texture and are excellent for evenly smoothing skin tones. If the proper shade is used, you may apply it without a foundation because it will blend easily into bare skin. Wand concealers provide a quicker, slightly denser coverage than liquid foundation, and they're absolutely fabulous for a fast repair. Some dry to a powder finish that's great for covering facial blemishes because the powder clings, enabling it to be longer wearing.

Pencil concealers effectively cover tiny imperfections such as broken capillaries, blemishes and other tiny flaws. You simply draw it on. With an exact color match, they can be pinpointed without blending. Pencil concealers are also terrific for fixing lip lines.

Oil-free compact concealer formulations are best used on the face to hide pimples and spots. They are usually of a longer-wearing, drier texture that won't irritate breakouts. Because of their wearability they are also effective for covering age spots and hyperpigmentation.

Highlight reflecting products thankfully are now available. They help to hide flaws but don't actually cover. Instead they have light-reflecting properties that refract light to help minimize shadowed areas. In other words, they highlight (bring out) recessed areas such as the dark shadows created by bags and wrinkles. You simply apply it to the shadowed area and it brightens it, making it appear less distinct. You should apply them sparingly. Too often they are confused with concealers, which they most definitely are not!

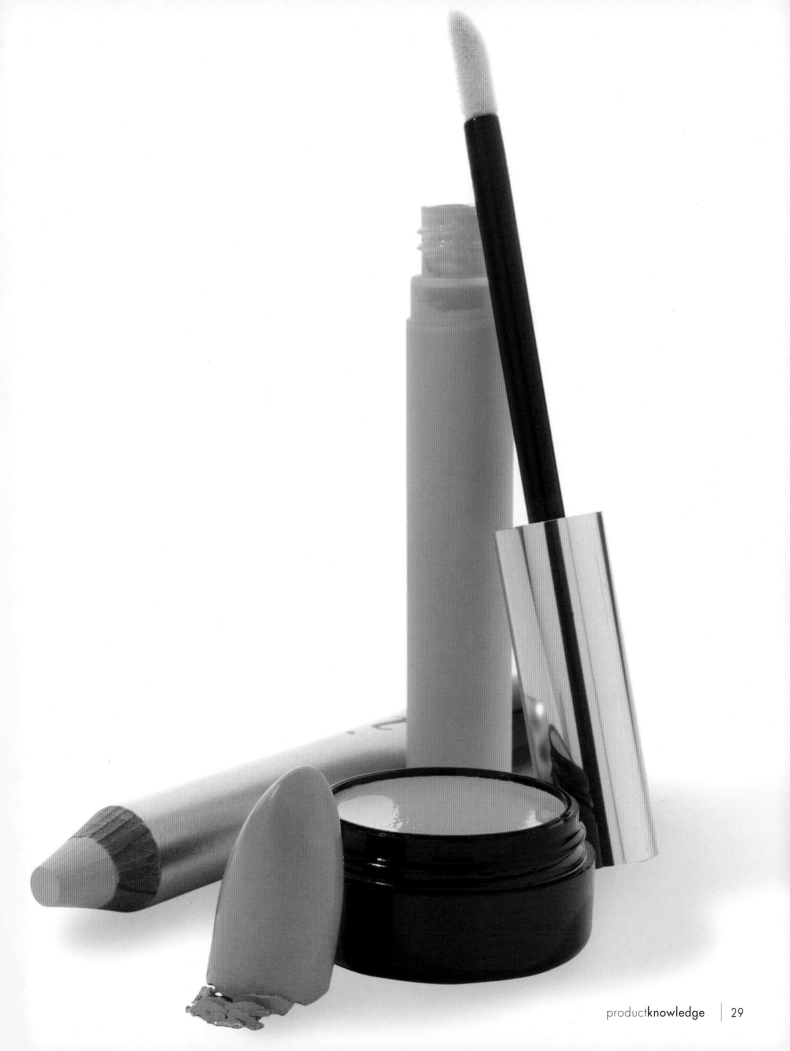

powder

provides staying power for your makeup—it won't last the day without it. It helps absorb the skin's natural oils to help control shine throughout the day. And it's the finishing step that helps your skin appear smooth and natural. You can even brush it on over a clean, moisturized face for a fresh, no-makeup look.

Most face powder is made from two bases: cornstarch and talcum. It basically comes in two forms, loose and pressed. Use a loose powder to set your makeup. It works best and lasts longest. Loose powder contains more oil absorbers than pressed, so it is the best choice for oily skin. Of course, if you travel, pressed powder is far more convenient to take along with you. Powder is an absolute must for oily skin. It absorbs extra oil from the skin and can be reapplied throughout the day. The finer a powder is milled, the higher the quality, so the less likely it is to cake on the skin. Finer-milled powders will feel more like velvet, whereas less-milled powders feel more gritty.

eyebrow

color is available in four formulas:

Pencil is the most precise and common way to define the brows. It usually has a slightly more waxy consistency than other makeup pencils to help it adhere better to the brows and last longer. If you prefer a brow pencil, make sure it is sharpened, because the sharper the point, the better the application.

Powder brow color is a matte, no-shimmer powder with a very high pigment content. It is usually applied with a brush and can be used to set brow crèmes and pencils to help them last longer. Powder provides the most natural look when filling in your brows.

Crème is the most dramatic looking and has the least natural appearance. It is a matte crème that is applied with a brush, and it's best to set it with powder so it will last. It gives you the most opaque coverage, which is sometimes needed.

Brow gel is basically a hair gel for the brows. It's great for unruly eyebrows because it helps keep the brows in place. Brow gels are available in tinted or clear formulas.

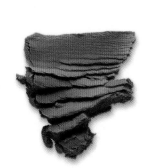

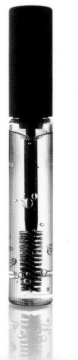

Tip:

Make sure the eyebrow pencil you choose is not too waxy, or it will be hard to apply evenly without looking harsh or fake.

mascara

generally comes in three formulas:

Thickening mascara coats each individual lash from root to tip with particles that add bulk to the lashes and help them to look thick and full.

Lengthening mascara contains plastic polymers that cling just to the tips of the lashes, making them appear longer.

Defining mascara coats the individual lashes, keeping them separated and defined. Defining mascara usually appears the most natural.

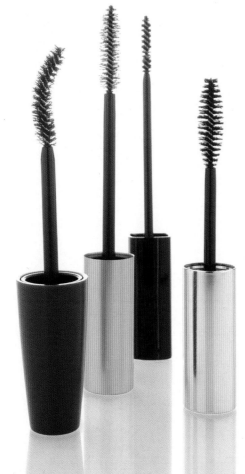

Most mascara is also available in a waterproof formula. However, unless you're susceptible to allergies that make your eyes water, you might not want a waterproof mascara because it's harder to remove and can damage delicate lashes. Also, women with sensitive eyes might want to stay away from waterproof because it is the most irritating of all formulas.

Most women don't realize that the mascara wand is just as important to the finished result of your lashes as the mascara formula.

There are four basic brush shapes.
• A crescent-shaped wand that helps keep your lashes curled as you apply your mascara.
• A fat, bristly wand that helps to thicken by coating each and every lash.
• A wand that looks much like a screw, and either has very short bristles or none whatsoever. It allows you to define your lashes by painting each one right down to the root.
• A double-tapered wand is a wand with smaller bristles at each end, tapering to fatter ones in the center. It works very nicely to define each thin, sparse lash while adding a little bulk.

It's always better to apply two thin coats of mascara rather than one thick, "clumpy" coat. I personally prefer thick, voluminous-looking lashes. I think they help define the eyes and they look so much more glamorous than thin, spidery-looking lashes.

eyeliner

comes in four basic formulas:

Liquid eyeliner is a colored liquid that is applied with a fine-tip brush. Liquid stays on the longest and looks the most dramatic. You can also find it in felt-tip pens or with a pointed, sponge-tip applicator. Liquid liner is a good choice to use with strip false eyelashes because it successfully conceals the band of the lash. Liquid eyeliner should only be applied along the top lashline, never along the bottom lashline, because it looks too harsh and unnatural.

Cake eyeliner is a pressed powder-like product that is applied with a damp brush. It will give you a similar effect to liquid eyeliner, but it's much easier to control.

Crème eyeliner is usually packaged in a pot and is applied using a damp brush. It will also give you a similar effect to liquid eyeliner. The fact that it dries much quicker makes it much easier to use without smearing it all over the place.

Pencil is the most commonly used eyeliner simply because it's the easiest to control. There are many pencil textures available. Some are drier and harder and some are creamier and glide on effortlessly. In the past, many women felt the need to soften their hard, dry pencils using a lighter or a match. Thankfully, most pencils now contain silicone that enables them to glide on smoothly and makes them easy to smudge and blend. The best choice is a pencil with just enough silicone to glide on easily, but not so much that it smears or travels. Make sure your pencil is at least water-resistant so it will stay put and not smudge.

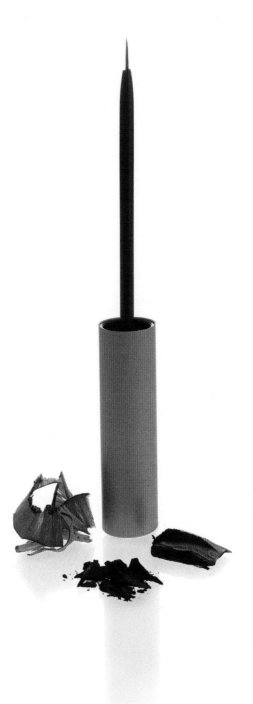

Tip:

Remember that sharpening your pencil often will make it easier to use.

eyeshadow

comes in various textures and finishes:

TEXTURES

Powder shadows come either loose or pressed. Both formulas vary from matte to shimmer and from iridescent to frosty. They are the most popular and the easiest to use because they blend so well. In most makeup lines, they offer the largest color choices in this texture.

Crème shadows are available in matte and shimmer. They are great for a wash of color across the whole lid. Be careful because many crème shadows can crease. However, there are some crème eyeshadows that dry to a powder finish. They work the best. You can also mix crème and powder eyeshadows together to increase the intensity of the shade.

Liquid usually comes in a shiny, metallic finish and it's actually the hardest to use. Since it doesn't blend easily you must be more precise, so it's best when applied with a brush. Liquid is usually used either as an eyeliner or applied close to the lashline for color intensity.

Pencil shadows are useful for around the eye because they are sharpened to a point and can be applied with such precision. When you've finished, you can simply smudge the line with your finger, a sponge-tip applicator, or a brush to create the effect you want.

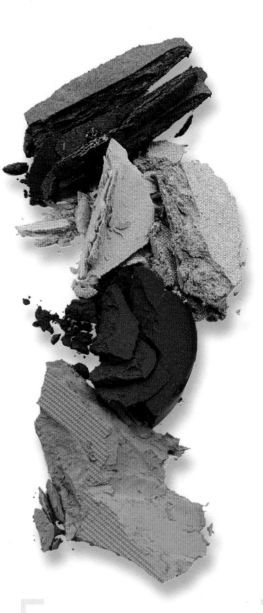

Tips:

For a more intense color, try using both powder and crème shadows together. Remember that powder on top of crème will hinder blending, but you still always begin with the crème. It contradicts the rule of crème-on-crème, powder-on-powder— but it works.

You can also use your powder shadow as eyeliner. Simply apply it wet or dry using a brush.

Some powder shadows are harder-pressed and more powdery, while others have a slightly creamy texture.

FINISHES

Matte is the best for creating a natural no-makeup look and is the best finish for midtone shades because of its natural appearance. It usually contains a higher level of color pigment and works really well for reshaping and defining the eye.

Shimmer shadows offer great, sheer coverage so that when you sweep on the color, you can still see the skin underneath. Shimmer shadows have a subtle sheen and give a hint of sparkle. They typically won't collect in fine lines, which makes them a perfect choice for mature skin. Light shimmer shadows work great for highlighting and bringing out recessed areas of the eyelid. Dark shimmer shadows are great for adding drama without being as harsh as deep-tone matte shades.

Frost shadows give much more opaque coverage and feature a white or silver sparkle. They usually come in fun, light pastel shades that work best on younger skin. Frosted shadows can easily sink into wrinkles and therefore do not work as well on mature skin.

Satin falls perfectly in between matte and shimmer. It's shinier than matte, but not nearly as shiny as a shimmer. A satin finish works well on all skin types, including mature skin.

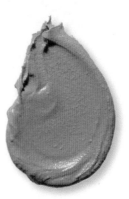

blush

usually comes in four different textures:

Powder blush is color pigment set in a powder base. Applied with a soft blush brush, it gives a dusting of color that works well with all skin types. It's the most popular type of blush because it's the easiest to control and use—and it's usually available in the widest range of shades. Powder blush is the best choice for oily skin.

Crème blush is color pigment set in a crème base. It has a fresh dewy finish that gives the face a luminous, natural glow. It is great on dry skin because it slides easily over the surface. It works best when applied before you powder because it will blend more easily. Unfortunately, if you have oily skin, crème blush is not your best choice because it won't wear well. And it doesn't work well on skin with large pores because it tends to accentuate them. It's great for those who don't need or want to wear foundation. Just apply it with your fingers or a sponge and work it into your skin.

Gel blush is basically made up of color pigments that are wrapped within silicone particles. It will smooth very nicely onto bare skin to create a pretty, sheer, translucent glow. That's not to say you can't use it with foundation; you can. Just make sure you apply it before you powder. It's long-lasting, looks very natural, and is easy to use. You can use your fingers or a sponge to apply it, then smooth it into the skin.

Liquid blush is actually a liquid that stains the skin. It's terrific for all skin types. It's applied like the gel blush, but is more difficult to work with because it must be blended quickly due to its staining quality. It's waterproof, so you can expect it to last all day. Just like crème blush or gel blush, you can use either a sponge or your fingers to apply and blend it into your skin.

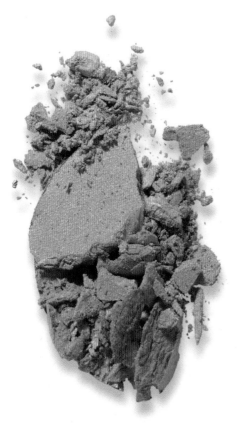

Tip:

If you're using powder blush directly on bare skin, be sure to powder your face first to prevent it from looking splotchy.

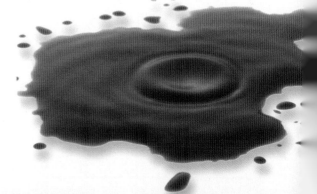

bronzer

is used to give the skin a warm, healthy glow. It usually comes in powder and crème formulas.

Powder bronzer, like powder blush, is the most popular because it's so easy to control and blend. It can come packaged in a variety of ways—pressed in a compact, loose in a tub, or even in a jar pressed into small balls or beads. Swept across strategic areas of the face with a brush, it can bring the skin to life.

Crème bronzer, like bronzing powder, is used to give the face a sun-kissed glow. You can find it in the form of a stick or even in compacts. It can be applied with your fingers or a sponge. It's great on dry skin, or when you don't want to wear foundation but want a little extra glow.

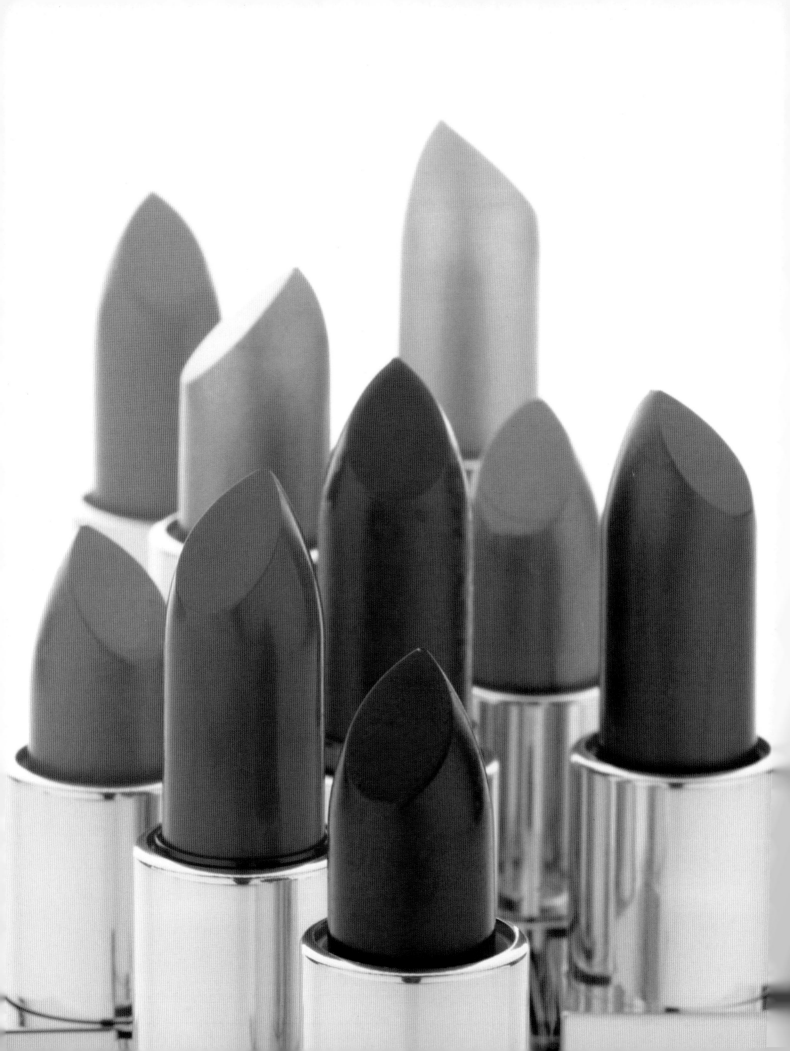

lipstick

is available in a variety of formulas:

Matte delivers sophisticated and intense full-coverage color that contains absolutely no shine. Because of its formulation it stays on longer, but it can be drying and may give your lips the feeling and appearance of being dehydrated. It is great in dark, intense shades because it stays put and won't smear, but it certainly does nothing to make the lips look younger or fuller.

Crème contains more emollients than matte lipstick and provides a full coverage of moist (though not shiny) color. Most cosmetic lines offer the largest selection in this formula because it is the most versatile and popular. It wears quite well without being as dehydrating as matte lipstick.

Frost provides a pale, shiny, metallic appearance. But because of the single color of sheen in the formula's ingredients, there is a tendency for the lips to appear a little dry. It usually gives very opaque coverage that is not wonderful for mature lips.

Sheer is actually a glossy, sheer color wash that allows the natural lips to show through because it is not formulated to cover opaquely. It's similar to a gel blush because it is simply pigments mixed with a gel. It lasts longer than a gloss, but not as long as a crème lipstick. It's terrific for a quick fix because, due to its sheerness, it doesn't have to be applied with precision.

Gloss is a lip color with extreme shine and moisture. It delivers a sheer layer of color that is going to need frequent reapplication. Although it doesn't last terribly long, gloss gives a fresh-and-alive look that's perfect for all age groups. Used correctly, it can make the lips look fuller and sexier. You'll find it packaged in a wand, tube, or pot.

Lip liner is a pencil that's used to define your lips. It helps correct lip shapes as well as prevent lip color from bleeding into fine lines. It can also be used over the entire lip, then topped with a color. Using a lip liner greatly improves the staying power of any lip color.

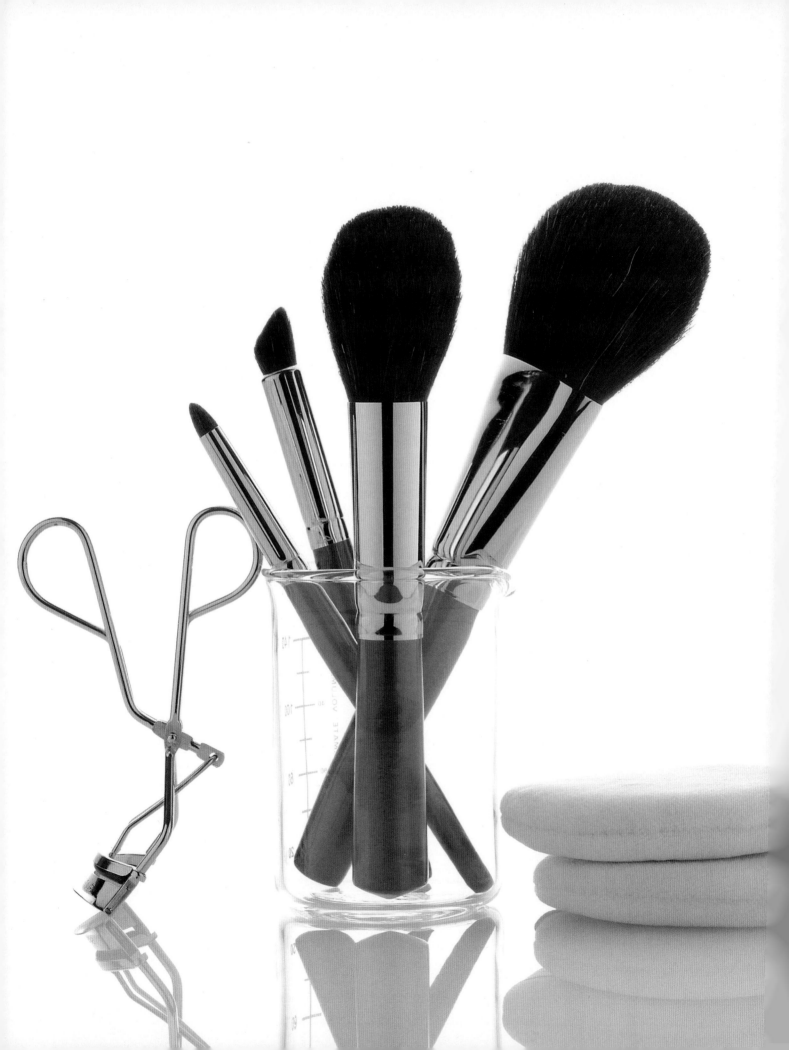

4

the tools

A painter selects the right brush to create the perfect stroke on a canvas, and so does a makeup artist—but in the case of the make-up artist, the canvas is skin. You can choose the right brush, too, with a little help from me. In this chapter, I've featured the best basic tools from my own brush collection to help you create the makeup effects you want. Remember: Makeup is like a work of art, an expression of your inner beauty. So experiment and have fun!

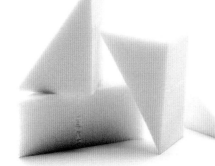

SPONGES

The most important thing to remember when selecting a sponge is that it should be made of a high-quality foam rubber so that it glides smoothly across your skin. It can be any shape you like—round, oval, triangular, or wedge—whatever feels the most comfortable in your hand. Use it for applying foundation and concealer or for blending.

POWDER PUFF

The best puffs are usually fluffy with a soft velour texture. It's a good idea to invest a little more and get a good-quality powder puff so you can launder it to keep it clean. Use it for applying pressed or loose powder.

EYELASH CURLERS

This tool is used to curl the lashes, which helps create the illusion of "opening up" the eyes. This is a must-have beauty tool for women of all ages.

There is now a choice for those that are afraid of crimp eyelash curlers. This curler (pictured below) will curl the most stubborn lashes because it uses heat and works with mascara. It is used after mascara to curl your lashes.

brushes

The following brushes are from my own collection of robert jones beauty makeup tools and organizational products.

EYEBROW

Eyebrow Brush #2. Shaped much like a mascara wand, this brush is very useful when trimming or grooming individual eyebrow hairs. Use it to help brush brows into place and to keep them perfectly shaped all day.

Angled Eyebrow Brush #1. This brush is perfectly angled to apply a crème or powder color to eyebrows. The firm bristles also work well for blending brow pencil lines.

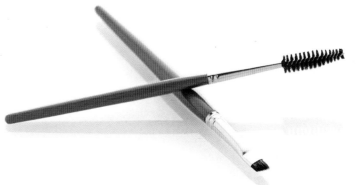

EYELINER

Fine Liner Brush #41. This flat, rectangular short-bristle brush is great for applying powder eyeliner at the base of the lashline or for pushing color right into the roots of the lashes to make lashes look thicker.

Liquid Liner Brush #42. This thin, pointed brush is perfect for applying liquid, crème, or cake eyeliner with precision.

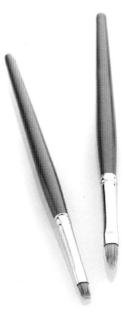

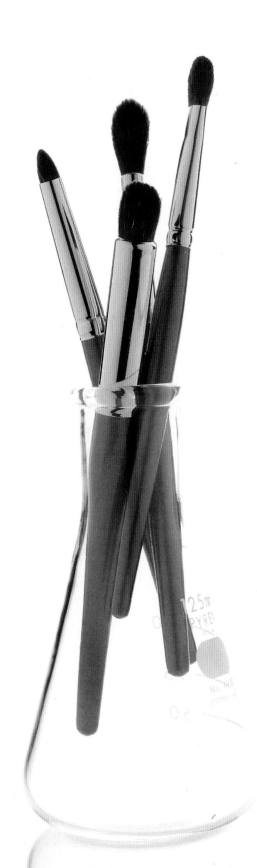

EYESHADOW

Eyeshadow Brush #13. This precision-style brush is perfect for applying your favorite shade of eye color along the lower lashline. Or use it to apply a very defined line of color into the crease of the eye.

Eyeshadow Brush #17. This firm, angled brush is great for applying a midtone color into the crease or for blending eyeshadow shades together.

Eyeshadow Brush #11. This large brush is great for applying midtone colors into the crease and for all-over blending of the eye colors—a must when you're wearing more than one eye color.

Eyeshadow Brush #12. This arched brush helps you precisely apply your most intense shade of eye color along your lashline and into the outer corners of the crease of your eyes.

BLUSH

Blush Brush #62. This full, soft brush is great for applying blush or bronzer. It's tapered toward the end to help you blend as you apply.

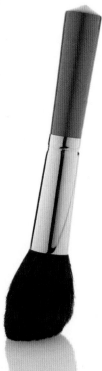

Foundation Brush #51. This large, smooth brush helps you evenly apply crème or liquid foundation onto the skin. Perfect for "end-of-the-day" touch-ups, it can help you create a smooth, even application over the foundation you are already wearing.

Jumbo Powder Brush #70. This big, fluffy brush is great for applying loose powder for a smooth, sheer and even application. It also is great for applying blush because it creates a soft, subtle effect.

Concealer Brush #50. This tapered brush is used for applying concealer with precision. It allows you to cover spots or flawed areas of the face without over-blending, so you actually conceal what you do not want to see.

Eyeliner Brush #40. The perfect brush to help you line and define your eyes with eyeshadow or to apply powder over your pencil eyeliner to create a more natural, subtle look.

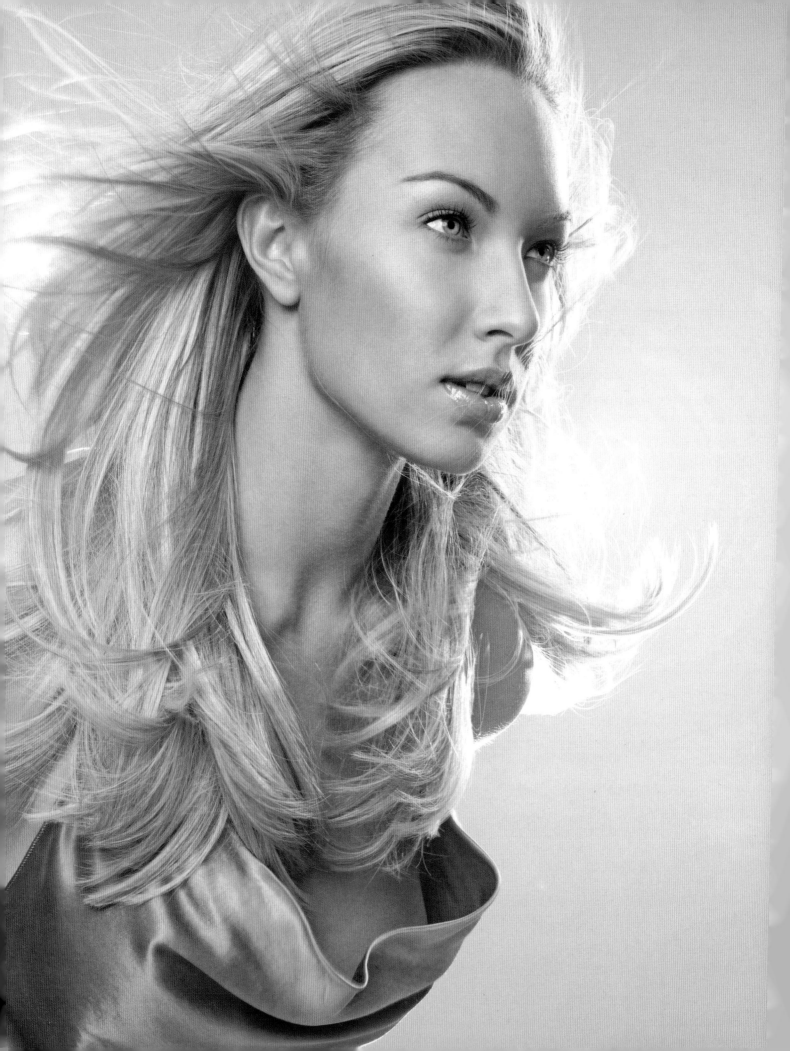

part two makeup and you

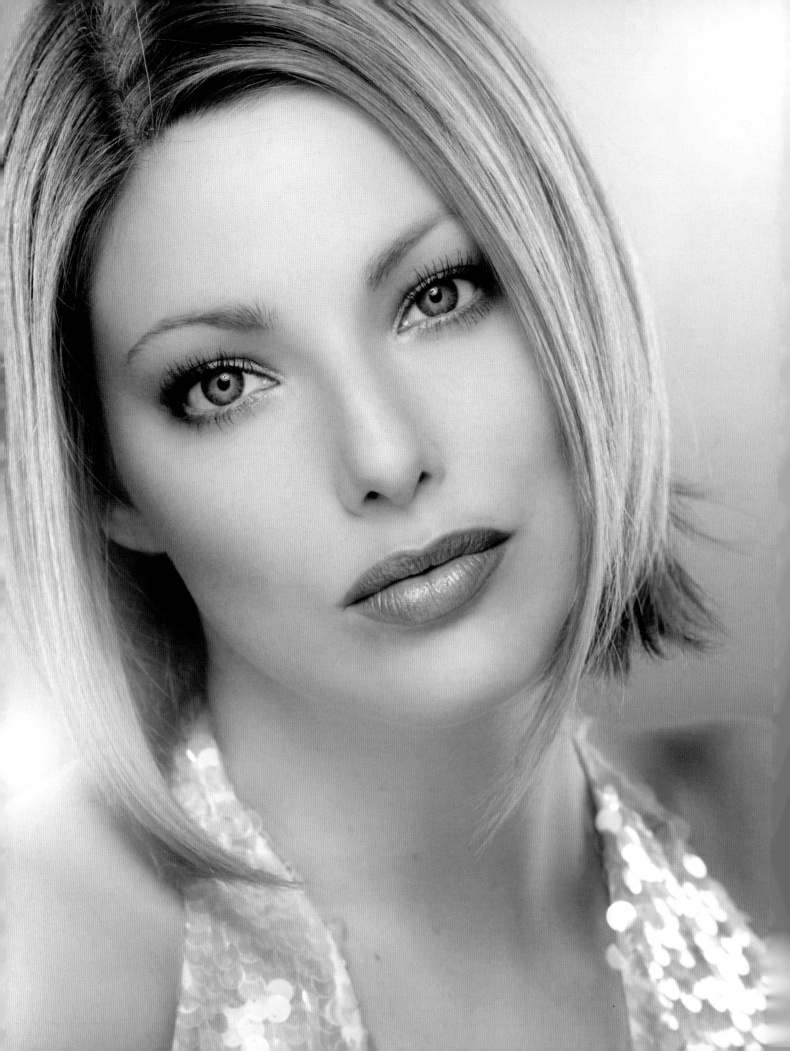

colorchoices

In this chapter, my goal is to help you make educated choices in selecting your color products. Choosing the correct shade of foundation is extremely important, since the wrong color can ruin the overall look of your makeup (and so can the wrong choice of eyeshadow, blush, or lipstick). Together, we can increase your chances of making the correct choices. Let's start the education process with a little foundation history.

All through the 1950s and '60s—really, until the late 1970s—women were told that it was correct to choose the opposite of their natural skin tone for their foundation color. For example, if your skin had olive undertones, you used a pink-based foundation, and if your undertones were pink, you used an orange-toned foundation.

And then in the 1980s, women were informed that this was all wrong, and they should match their skin's exact undertone. So if you had pink undertones, your foundation color had to be pink-based. If your undertones were olive, you put on an olive-toned foundation—well, you get the picture.

Then finally in the 1990s, the cosmetic industry discovered that yellow undertones, instead of being undesirable, actually made the skin look the most alive and natural. Yellow is the one color that everyone has in their skin, from the very lightest complexion to the darkest. It's just that some people have other colors in their skin as well, such as shades of red or brown. Almost everyone looks better with some yellow in their foundation. It counteracts the skin tones you don't want to see and enhances the tones that you do want to see.

Thankfully now there are more and more innovations in products than ever before, so that with most good-quality foundations, you don't even know that they are there. They are sheer, yet totally cover and give you flawless-looking skin. It is still absolutely essential that you make the best choice for you so let's talk about how to make that perfect choice. We already discussed all the different types, now let's discuss making the right shade choice.

SKIN TONE

Let's try to make this simple.

There are approximately fifteen levels of depth to the skin. "Depth" is the lightness or darkness of your skin, with Level 1 being very pale (porcelain) and Level 15 being very dark (ebony). When choosing foundation, there are two factors to consider. First, you want it to match the depth level of your skin —i.e., the lightness or darkness of your skin. Starting on page 52, I have provided photos of eight before-and-after makeovers to show you examples of skin tones, ranging from light to dark. These photos will help you understand the link between the depth level of skin and foundation.

Second, you must match it to the undertone of your skin. The majority of women have "warm" undertones. In my opinion, warmer skin always looks more youthful. A very small number of women have truly "cool" undertones. They have dark hair, pale skin and light eyes. (Think Snow White.) Even if you start out cool, the minute you go out into the sun, you become warm. If you come from certain backgrounds—Italian, Hispanic, Asian, or African-American—you're warm. If you have brown or green eyes, you're warm. If you are able to tan well, you're definitely warm.

One of the biggest makeup mistakes women make is thinking they have cool undertones when they don't. That's why it's always important to conduct a "stripe test" to make sure you're wearing the right foundation to match your skin depth level. On page 56, you'll learn how to properly conduct a stripe test.

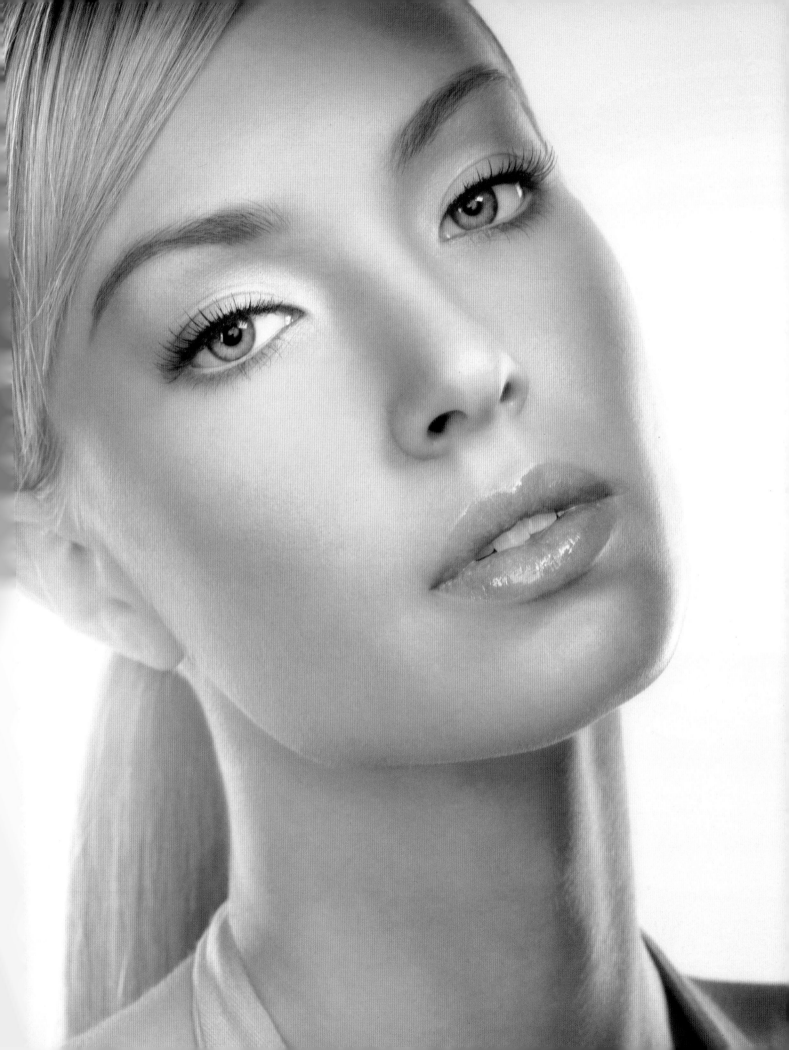

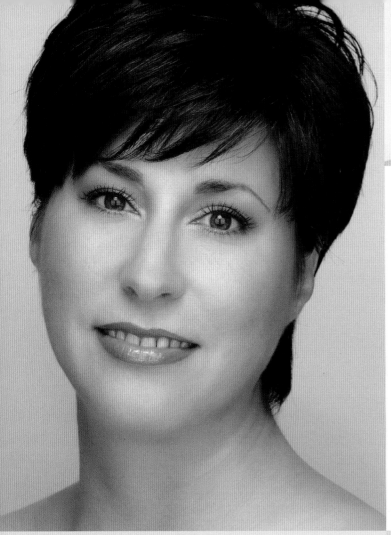

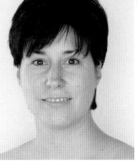

rhonda shasteen

FACE SHAPE: pear
EYE SHAPE: close-set
SHADOWS: Highlight: shimmer flesh
              Midtone: matte taupe
              Contour: shimmer golden brown
OBJECTIVE: To give the illusion of a more oval-shaped face. To visually pull the eyes apart.
APPLICATION: Contoured the jawline and cheeks to minimize their width. Highlighted the forehead to create the illusion of more width. Highlighted the inner corner of eyelids to visually push the eyes apart. Defined the outer corners of the eyes with the deepest shadow.

sherril steinman

FACE SHAPE: pear
EYE SHAPE: hooded
SHADOWS: Highlight: shimmer beige
              Midtone: matte dark taupe
              Contour: matte dark brown
OBJECTIVE: To give the illusion of a more oval-shaped face. To minimize the hooded appearance of the eyelids, making her eyes appear more open.
APPLICATION: Contoured the jawline and cheeks to minimize their width. Highlighted the forehead to create the illusion of more width. Using midtone and contour colors, applied, then blended them to the hooded area, giving the illusion that the area recedes.

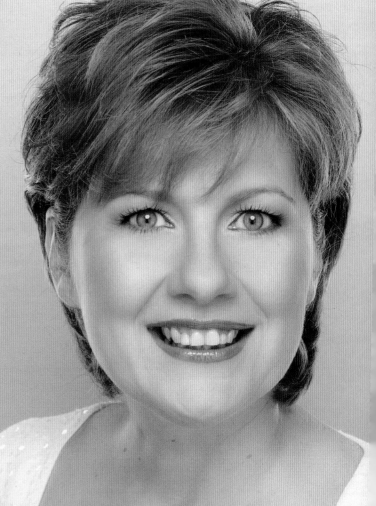

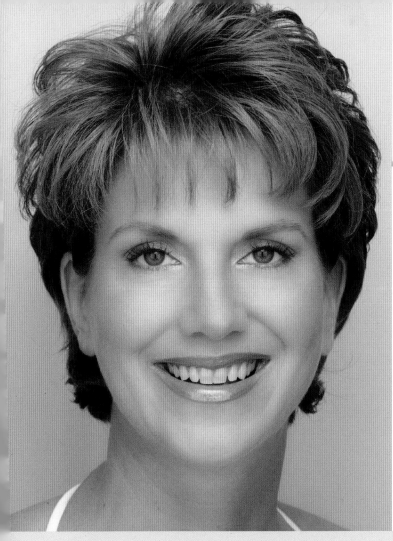

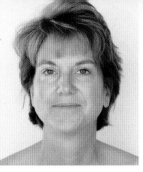

linda bird

FACE SHAPE: pear
EYE SHAPE: basic
SHADOWS: Highlight: shimmer beige
               Midtone: matte taupe
               Contour: shimmer golden brown
OBJECTIVE: To give the illusion of a more oval-shaped face.
APPLICATION: Contoured the jawline and cheeks to minimize their width. Highlighted forehead to create the illusion of more width. Highlighted the eyelid to brighten the eye, then concentrated on defining the crease and the lash line.

michelle boye

FACE SHAPE: square
EYE SHAPE: wide-set
SHADOWS: Highlight: shimmer beige
               Midtone: matte dark taupe
               Contour: shimmer golden brown
OBJECTIVE: To give the illusion of a more oval-shaped face. To make it appear as if the eyes are closer together.
APPLICATION: Contoured hairline and jawline to soften the "four corners" of the face. Highlighted down the center of the forehead, nose and chin. Applied a darker midtone to the inside hollow of her eyes to visually pull the eye placement closer together.

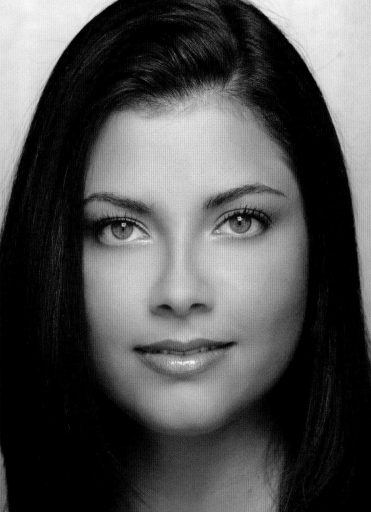

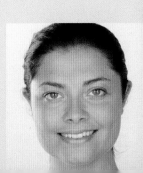

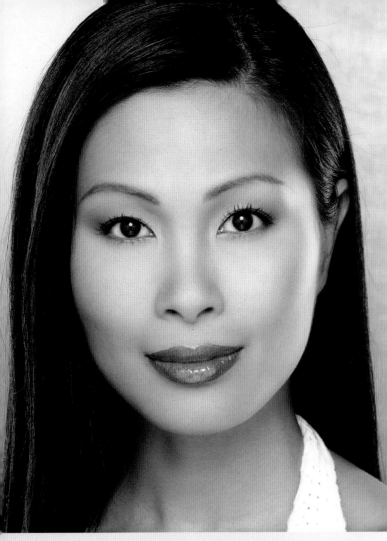

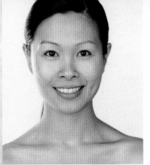

eleanor simon

FACE SHAPE: oval
EYE SHAPE: hooded
SHADOWS: Highlight: shimmer beige
   Midtone: matte dark taupe
   Contour: shimmer golden brown
OBJECTIVE: To minimize the hooded appearance of the eyelids, causing her eyes to appear more open and alive.
APPLICATION: Applied midtone and contour color to the hooded area of the lids to help them recede and open up the eyes. Subtly layered color, starting with one layer of midtone, then following with additional layers to help the hooded area appear to recede naturally.

lydia duron

FACE SHAPE: pear
EYE SHAPE: hooded
SHADOWS: Highlight: shimmer beige
   Midtone: matte dark taupe
   Contour: matte dark brown
OBJECTIVE: To give the illusion of a more oval-shaped face. To minimize the hooded appearance of her eyelids, causing her eyes to look more open and alive.
APPLICATION: Contoured the jawline and cheeks to minimize their width. Highlighted the forehead to help create width. Subtly layered color on the hooded areas of the eyes to help minimize them and open up the eyes.

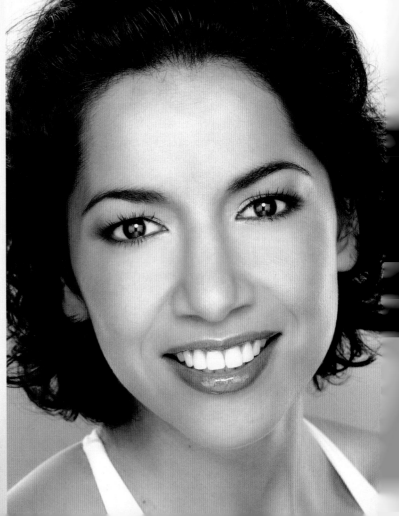

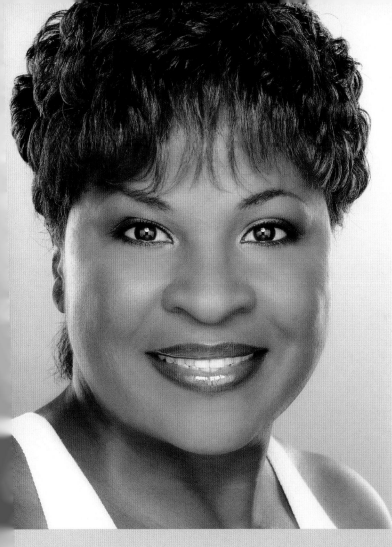

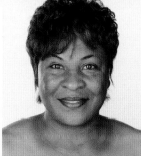

sonja hunter mason

FACE SHAPE: round
EYE SHAPE: wide-set
SHADOWS: Highlight: shimmer gold
Midtone: matte mahogany
Contour: dark burgundy
OBJECTIVE: To give the illusion of a more oval shaped face. To even out skin tone and brighten areas to add life to the face.
APPLICATION: Using multiple shades of foundation, evened out skin tone, then highlighted areas with a golden-orange face powder to give life to the skin. Softly sculpted her cheeks, jaw, and temples. Highlighted the lid and contoured the inside hollow of her eyes to visually pull them closer.

alischia butler

FACE SHAPE: square
EYE SHAPE: basic
SHADOWS: Highlight: shimmer gold
Midtone: matte mahogany
Contour: dark burgundy
OBJECTIVE: To give the illusion of a more oval-shaped face. To even out skin tone and brighten areas to add life to the face.
APPLICATION: Using multiple shades of foundation, evened out the slight skin discoloration. The main goal was to brighten her face, which was achieved by using a golden-orange face powder to highlight areas. Contoured hairline and jaw to soften the "four corners" of the face.

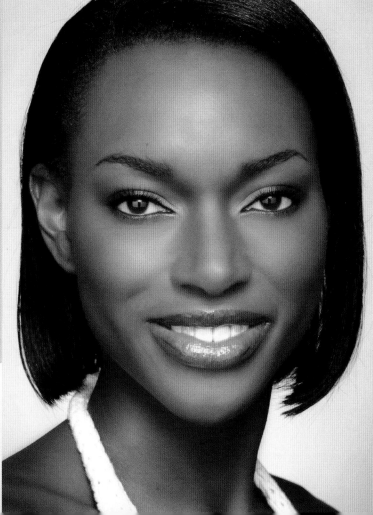

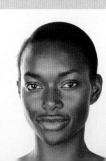

foundation

The best way to choose a foundation color is to conduct
a stripe test. Here are a few fast rules to follow so you
won't "flunk." Always conduct your stripe test in
natural light. Start with three different foundation
shades to compare and contrast. (The area where you
will test the shades will vary depending on your skin
tone.) Finally, if the shade you choose is the best
match with your neck color, you will pass the stripe
test with flying colors.

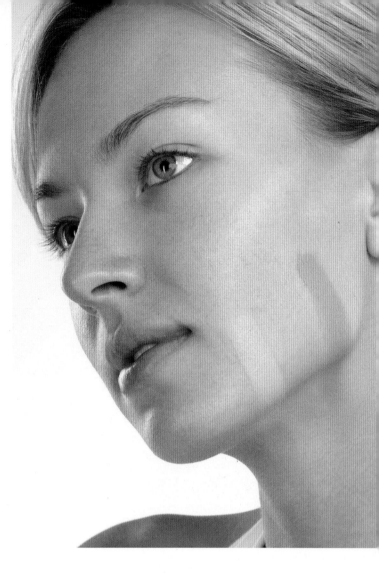

IVORY AND BEIGE

If you have ivory or beige skin tones, conduct the stripe
test from jaw to neck to get a true match to the neck.
Women with these skin types tend to have redness in
their faces, but not in their necks, so it's important to get
a true match. Start by applying three stripes of the different foundation shades from your jaw to your neck and
wait a few minutes to see if the oils in your skin change
the color pigments. Select the one that most closely
matches your neck.

BRONZE AND EBONY

Women with bronze and ebony skin tones should stripe-test from the cheek area to the jaw area, because some women with these skin tones have "facial masking," or lighter skin on the interior of the face and darker skin on the outer edges of the face. Start by applying three stripes of the different foundation shades extending from your cheek to your jaw area, and wait a few minutes to see if the oils in your skin change the color pigments.

If you have any degree of facial masking, I suggest using my technique of applying two shades of foundation to perfect your skin tone: one shade to brighten your skin, and another to deepen it. Turn to page 84 to find out why two shades are better than one when it comes to facial masking and how to apply them.

CHOOSE YELLOW OVER PINK

As I said before, a shade of yellow foundation complements almost any skin tone. The only time pink is a better choice is if you have pink undertones in your neck as well as your face, which is very rare. Most women with pink in their faces do not have it in their necks. Pink foundation on top of a pink face can become red—and no one wants a red face. Foundations and powders with pink hues actually age the skin and make it appear unnatural, yet many mature women choose pink to give their faces more color. Remember that color should be provided by your blush and lipstick—not by your foundation and powder.

Yellow foundations can actually counteract skin conditions such as rosacea and broken capillaries. Women with these conditions or with ruddy skin tones often feel that yellow foundations look too yellow because they're used to seeing all the red in their faces. Give it time! Your skin will start to absorb the foundation and work with it better, and your eye will get used to seeing the red neutralized. You'll soon notice a more even, natural skin tone.

In contrast, many women with yellow in their skin will try to counteract that by choosing a pink foundation. This is never a good choice. You should embrace and enhance the yellow tones in your skin to make it appear younger, more fresh, and alive.

Women with ebony skin should match the undertones in their skin exactly because they are so distinct and noticeable. They can range all the way from golden-orange to true brown. Keep in mind that it is always a good idea to brighten (not lighten) ebony skin. Intense golden-orange tones work well for brightening ebony skin.

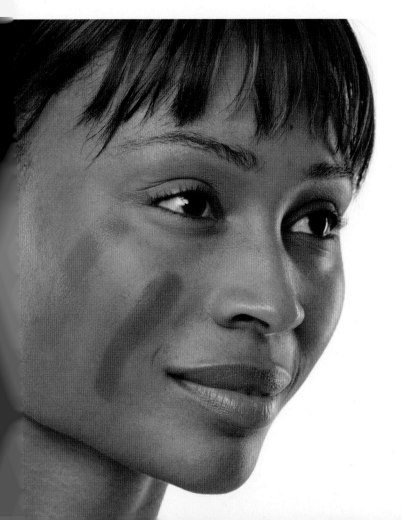

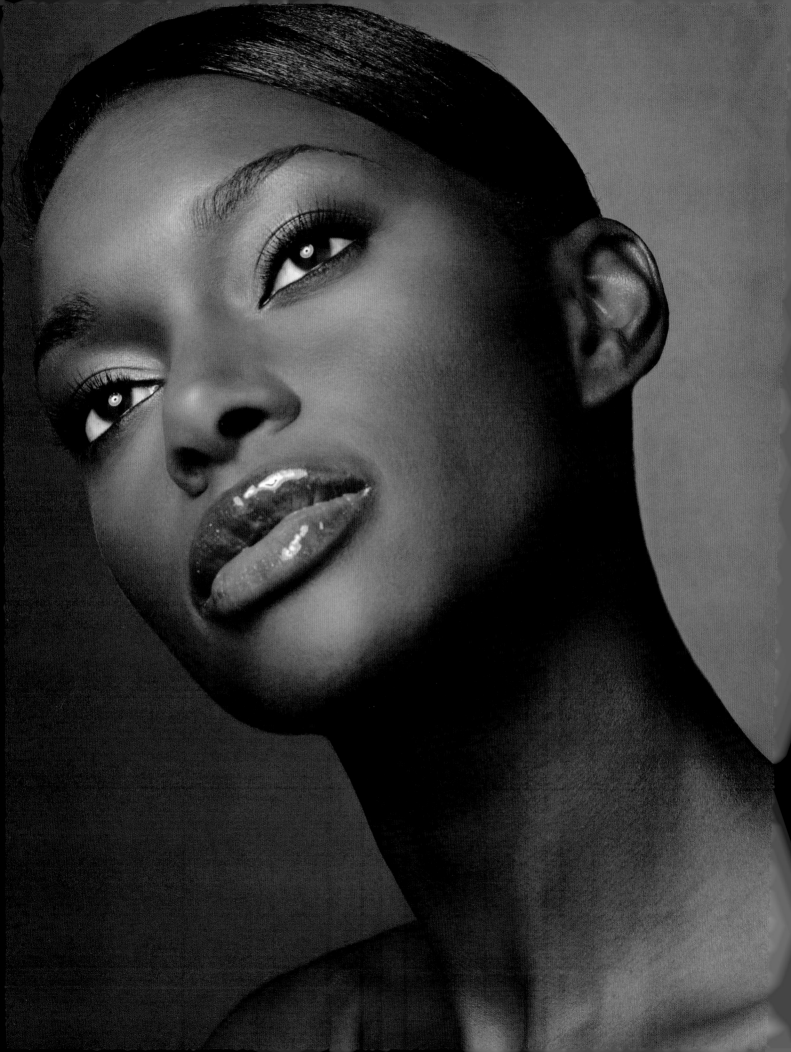

concealer

IVORY AND BEIGE

You can get a lot of mileage out of concealers with yellow undertones. Yellow is the best color choice because it works to counteract most skin imperfections, including the purple of undereye circles, the brown of age spots, and any ruddiness or red in the complexion. The more severe the imperfection—such as a port-wine stain or extremely dark circles—the more yellow you will need in your concealer.

BRONZE AND EBONY

On bronze and ebony skin, a golden-orange concealer for lighter to medium skin tones works wonderfully. For really deep tones of ebony, a warm-brown concealer usually covers best.

powder

IVORY AND BEIGE

As with foundation and concealer, a face powder with yellow or neutral undertones is usually the best choice. I never recommend using a face powder with pink undertones because it can make the skin appear artificial and older. Your goal should be to find a neutral shade of powder to match your foundation exactly. Or, if you want to warm up your skin or correct imperfections, you should choose a powder with yellow undertones.

BRONZE AND EBONY

Women with bronze and ebony skin tones should use a powder with golden-orange undertones to brighten and freshen the skin to a beautiful glow. The darker the skin, the more likely that you should use a powder with warm brown undertones to give the skin a glowing, natural look. Dark bronze and ebony skin tones also should choose a loose powder with a hint of shimmer to it. This will help absorb any oils in the skin and keep it looking fresh and dewy. Loose powders with a matte finish can make bronze and ebony skin appear very flat and ashy.

One more important point about powder: Translucent powder is not invisible (transparent), though the two words are easy to confuse. It is less opaque than other powders, but it is not colorless and can often appear unnatural, especially on dark beige and olive skin tones. It's always best to choose a powder that is an appropriate match for your skin tone, or one that brightens your skin. The one time translucent powder is helpful is when powdering areas that have been heavily concealed.

eye color	liner	shadow
blue	warm brown taupe	rich warm browns warm taupes soft peaches
green	red-brown taupe purple	golden browns warm taupes deep purples soft peaches soft violets
brown	rich brown charcoal taupe purple	golden brown blue green light mahogany charcoal purple
grey	charcoal deep brown	charcoal cool brown purple

eyeshadow

The most important thing to remember about choosing eyeshadow is…YOU! Look at the color of your eyes. Consider your skin tone. Then select a shade that will bring out the natural color of your eyes. Your goal is to make your eye color "pop" or stand out—not compete with, or diminish your natural color in any way.

The chart on the opposite page can help you select shades that will enhance your eyes. Notice there is no blue shade suggested for blue eyes or green shadows for green eyes. The key is to select a color that's the opposite of your own eye color. For example, the opposite of blue eyes is a warm shade of brown, or tawny, or golden shades.

Brown-eyed girls have it best. They can experiment with a variety of colors and still enhance their natural eye color. So play to your heart's content with purple, green, gold, or brown. Any color looks beautiful around brown eyes.

If you are wondering why you do not see a category on the chart for hazel eyes, it is because they are not just one color. Hazel eyes are either a mixture of blue and green or green and brown. So depending on which you have you can place them in two different categories. If you have blue and green hazel eyes you can choose shades from the blue or the green category. If you have green and brown hazel eyes you can choose shades from the green category. So it is up to you to decide, don't be scared to experiment.

Skin tone is another thing to consider. Women with dark ebony skin should not choose an eyeshadow that is too white or light. Likewise, women with fair, pale skin might want to stay away from eyeshadows that are too dark. Subtle, natural colors look better than dramatic contrasting shades—especially during the daytime.

Finally, you do not have to match your eye makeup to your clothing. Makeup is an accessory to you, just like your clothing. Makeup is *not* an accessory to your clothing. Matching your makeup colors to your clothes can sometimes wash you out and may not always flatter your best features. Choose what looks best on you. Apply your makeup as if you're wearing white, just like the models in this book. That way your real beauty can shine through and not take a back seat to your clothing or eye makeup.

EYELINER

No matter what your eye color is, choose neutral shades of eyeliner, such as taupe, black, or brown, to shape and define your eyes. Colored eyeliners can help draw attention to your eyes by making the color "pop," but I recommend saving them for when you want to make a more dramatic makeup statement.

eyeshadow palette

To show you how simple but versatile makeup
can be, I chose a basic eyeshadow palette (shown
in the chart on the opposite page) to create every
before-and-after look in parts one, two, and three.
I believe that, with this palette, any woman can
look beautiful, regardless of her eye shape or whether
she has an ivory, beige, bronze, or ebony skin tone.
Notice that the shades fall into three categories:
highlight, midtone, and contour. Using these three
depth categories of color helps give shape to your
eyelids. To learn more about this simple application
technique, turn to page 129.

shimmer	flesh	highlight	
shimmer	beige	highlight	
shimmer	gold	highlight	
matte	sand	highlight	
matte	taupe	midtone	
matte	rose	midtone	
matte	dark taupe	midtone	
matte	caramel	midtone	
matte	mahogany	midtone	
shimmer	golden brown	contour	
matte	dark brown	contour	
matte	burgundy	contour	
matte	black	contour	

blush

Blush can brighten your face and make it positively glow. The trick is to find a blush color that's natural and neutral but still brightens and adds life to the skin. The best way to decide what shade to wear is to take a quick jog around the block and see what natural color your cheeks blush.

For ivory or light beige skin tones, a blush with soft pink undertones is usually your best choice. As you mature, you may want to switch to a blush with peach undertones instead of pink to help your skin appear brighter and fresher. The color peach is a mature woman's best friend. It can warm and enhance the skin, while pink often appears ashy and artificial on the skin as it ages.

Women with olive skin tones should use blush with warm undertones that have a richness or intensity so the color shows up on the skin, such as tawny shades of cinnamon or sunny copper. If you have ebony or bronze skin tones, you should also choose a blush with warm undertones, such as apricot or paprika, to give your skin a nice warm glow that appears natural. For a more dramatic look, women with bronze and ebony skin tones can choose a blush with brick red or red-brown undertones for more intense color on the skin. The very best choice for all skin tones is a blush that looks soft and natural and appears to give you a glow from within.

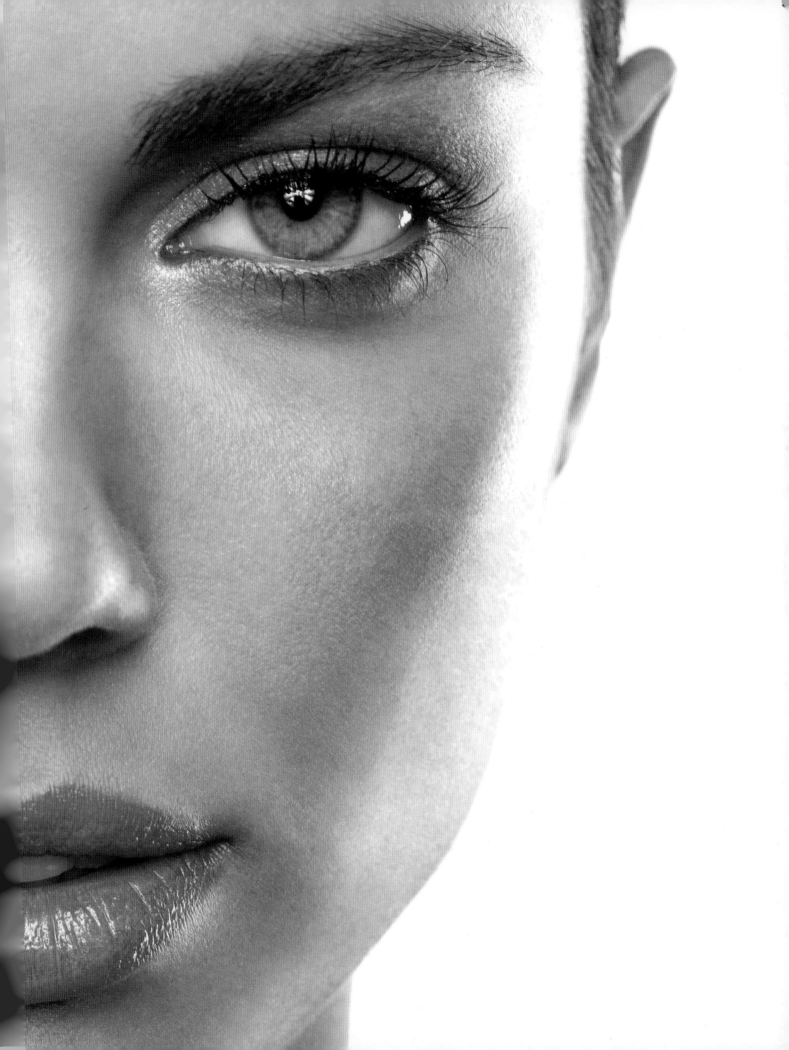

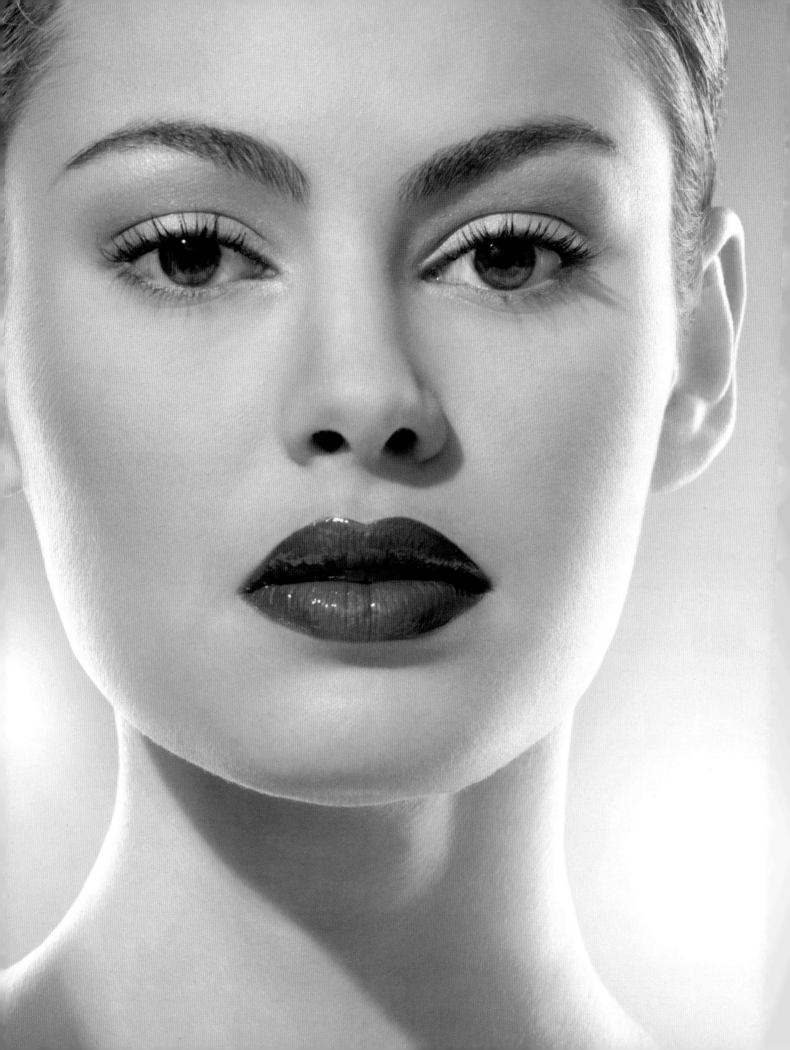

lips

When it comes to choosing a lip color, size definitely matters. If you have full, beautiful lips, you can wear darker shades as long as they complement your skin tone. Wear lighter shades of lip color on thin lips to make them look fuller. The chart found here can help you find the perfect lip shades for you.

Skin tone is very important to consider before choosing a lip color. Women with ivory skin tones should not wear chocolate brown lipstick, for example, because it can age you and appear unnatural— a woman with ivory skin would never have that much brown in her lips. Women with bronze skin tones should not wear pale, frosty lip shades, because they can make lips appear ashy and artificial.

Here are two more things to remember: Dark lip colors age you faster than any other makeup product. And warmer, more colorful lipstick choices always make you appear younger, because they bring out the warm tones in your skin and add life to your face. So lighten up and have fun with your lip color! The beauty of wearing lipstick is that it adds life to your face and makes it appear more healthy and alive.

skin tones	lipsticks
fair	glossy transparent pinks light peach honey beige
medium	medium pinks light mocha caramel delicate red medium apricots tangy peach
olive	strong red deep rose berry toffee mahogany dark apricots brown red
ebony	deep brownish red deep berry deep fuchsia golden beige

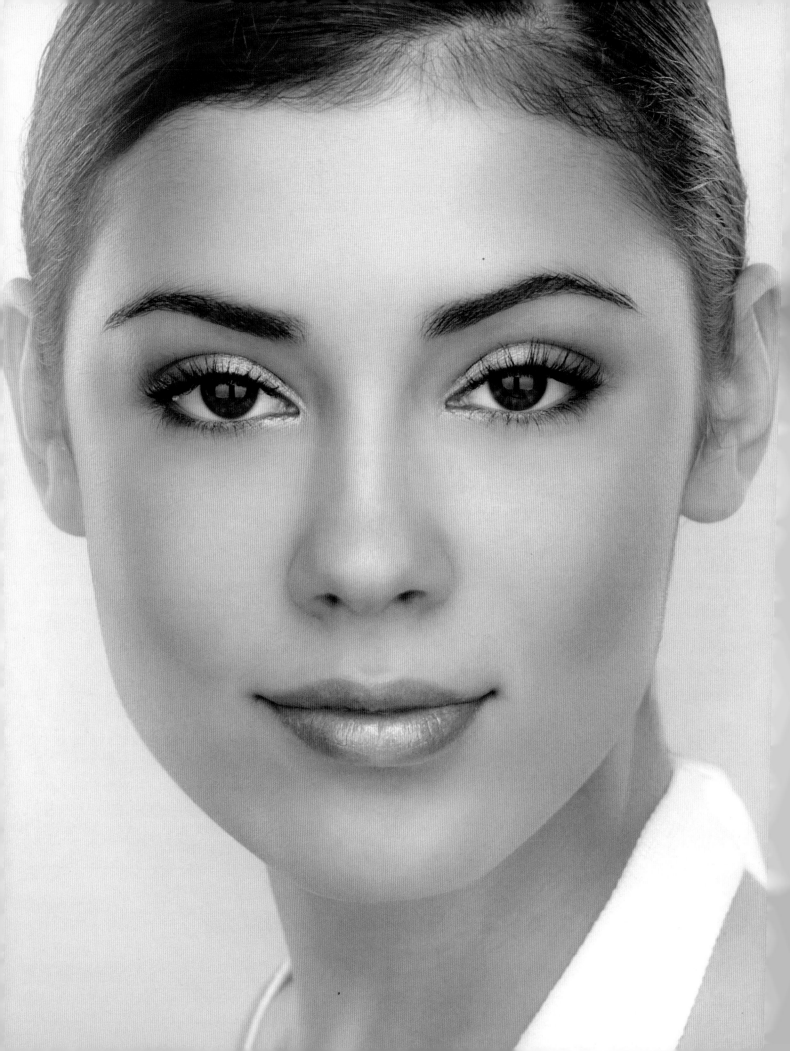

canvas**prep**

Getting a flawless finish begins with a few simple tricks up front. From perfectly arched brows to skin that's been easily prepped for makeup application, you'll find that it doesn't take a lot to get results that everyone will see.

brow attack

Well-groomed eyebrows are a beauty must. You should embrace your natural brow shape, because no matter how much you tweeze, you cannot turn them into something they are not. Some brows naturally curve into a gentle arch; others grow straight across. The only way you can turn a straight brow into a curved one is by tweezing it away completely and drawing in a new one. But do not try this at home—or anywhere else! You'll find a simple, better way to find the best shape for your brows on the next few pages.

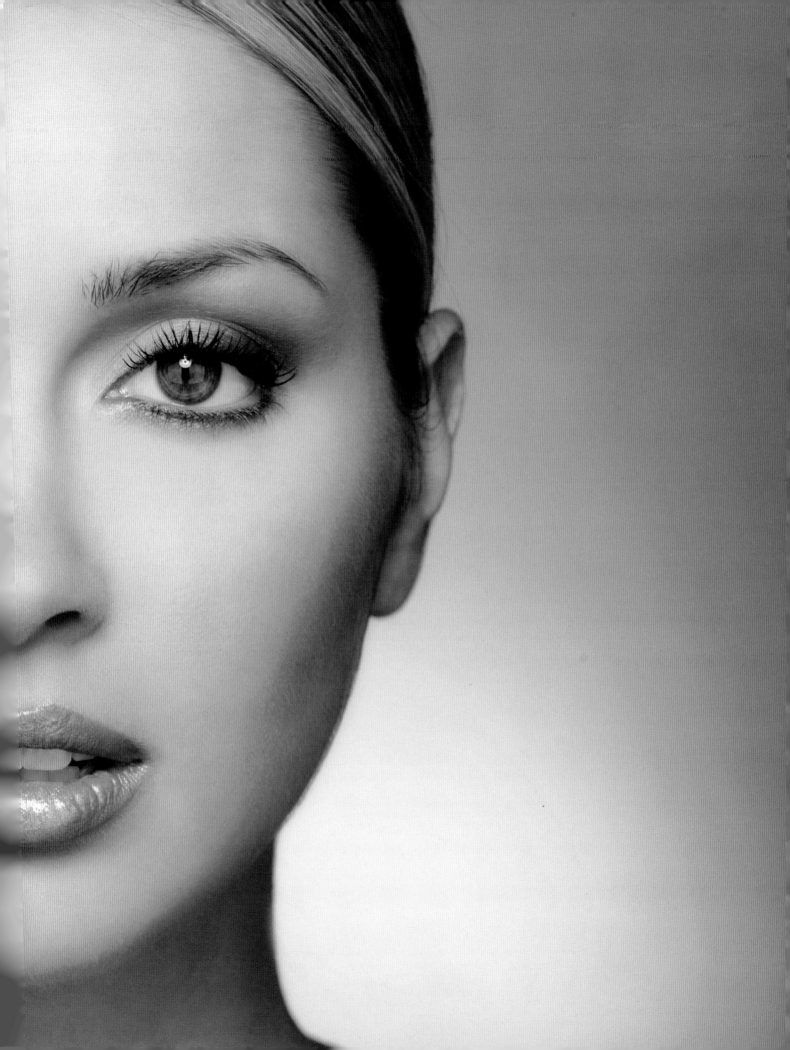

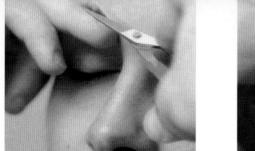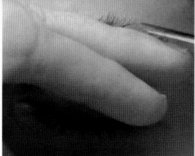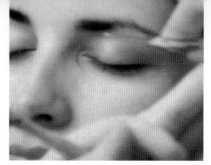

Before we begin, gather your tools together. You will need a pair of tweezers, a brow brush, a small pair of scissors, and a white eye pencil.

Now let's evaluate your brows.

First, are they too dense? Eyebrows that are too dense can be softened either by trimming them or lightening the color.

To trim them, simply brush them up and snip any stray hairs that extend past the upper brow line. Next, brush them down and snip any unruly hairs that extend past the lower brow line.

Often, brow hairs are actually longer than they appear because the tips of the hairs are light in color and when they reach a certain length they tend to curl. By trimming them, you trim away some of the density and that slight curl so that the hairs lay down more neatly.

It's important to remember that if you need to trim your brows, it should be done before you start to tweeze. Otherwise you might ruin your brow line by tweezing away hairs that should have stayed but were simply too long.

Are your brows too pale, or are they speckled with gray? If they are, you might choose to have them tinted. Tinting will help define them and alleviate the need for eyebrow makeup.

Now it's tweeze time.

The best time to tweeze your brows is after a steamy shower. It's a lot less painful because your pores are already open. Try to tweeze in natural light. You can see what you're doing much better.

After plucking a couple of hairs from one brow, move to the other, then back and forth a few hairs at a time to preserve the symmetry. Always tweeze in the same direction as the hair grows or the hair might not grow back properly.

A great trick when preparing to tweeze is to use a white eye pencil to sketch a pattern outline (a template of sorts) of the shape you want your brow to be. This is an excellent way to get a preview of the end result before you actually do the tweezing. It's then a simple matter to remove only the hairs that are covered in white.

Tip:

Take care not to overdo it, because sparse brows, especially on a mature face, make the face look older.

You can wax unwanted hairs, but be aware that the hairs may not grow back correctly because wax is pulled off in the opposite direction to the hairs' growth. Also, a warning: Waxing repeatedly may eventually give a crepe-like appearance to the skin.

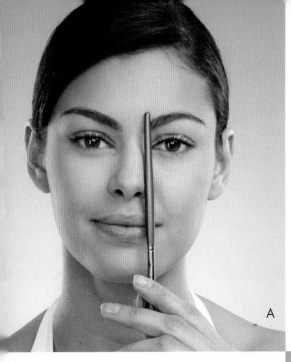

HOW DO YOU DETERMINE WHERE TO START?

Here's how to make the perfect eyebrow take shape. Locate three pivotal points along your brow line by following this quick exercise:

Point A. Hold a pencil or the handle of a brush vertically against the side of your nose, noticing where it meets the brow. That is where your brow should begin.

Point B. Hold the pencil against your nostril and move it diagonally across the outer half of the iris of your eye. Notice where the pencil meets the brow. This is the best place for the peak of your arch. If you tweeze from Point A to Point B, tapering the line slightly thinner toward the peak, you will create the ideal shape for your brow.

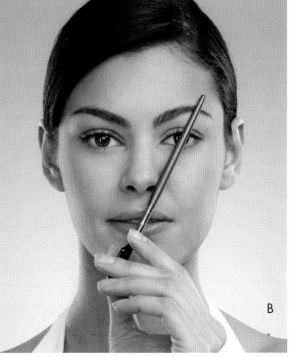

Point C. Again, place the pencil against your nostril and extend it diagonally to the outer corner of your eye. Where it meets the brow is the best place for your brow to end. If you tweeze from Point B to Point C, tapering the line even thinner, you will create the best brow shape for your face.

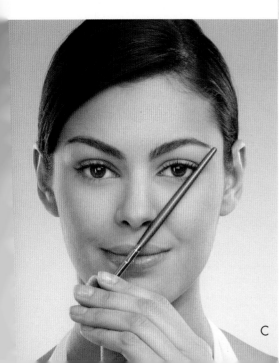

moisturizer

Moisturizing is an important step that helps your foundation go on smoothly and evenly.

Make sure to begin with a freshly washed face, then apply your moisturizer. It's best applied to a damp face because it goes on more evenly. Moisturizer evens the skin's porosity and is most effective when it's left to absorb for a few minutes before you apply your makeup. You can use a light moisturizer or a heavy one; just make sure you choose the right one for your particular skin type.

• Moisturizers for normal skin are usually light to help even out any dry areas.

• Moisturizers for dry skin are usually higher in emollients and are richer.

• Moisturizers for sensitive skin are fragrance- and irritant-free.

• Moisturizers for oily skin are extremely light and won't clog pores. Many have oil-absorbing properties in them that actually help control the oil. Oily skin needs moisturizer, because it can often be over-dried by cleansers. The body is so smart, it actually produces more oil to compensate for the over-dryness, which only makes the complexion appear greasier. A light moisturizer keeps oily skin from producing more oil and can help even out its porosity.

Tip:

Never apply moisturizer to the eyelids before your eyeshadow because it will cause it to crease and not last as long.

Moisturizing your lips before applying lip color will help it go on more smoothly.

primer

Primer is an optional makeup step that can do wonders for your skin's appearance. It helps your foundation go on more evenly and makes it last longer. Primer sometimes contains light-reflecting properties that reflect light and help diminish the appearance of some of your small flaws. So it can help your skin appear more perfect and help it stay fresh-looking all day. It also helps prevent your foundation color from altering due to your skin's natural oils, because it creates a barrier between those natural oils and your foundation. Simply apply it on top of your moisturizer before you apply your foundation.

exfoliate

You should exfoliate your lips regularly to keep your lip texture smooth and soft. A great time to do this is right after you shower. Just apply a generous amount of lip balm and wait a few minutes for it to absorb. Using a soft-bristle toothbrush, brush your lips vigorously then reapply more lip balm. If you prefer, you can use a towel to rub your lips instead of a brush. Whichever method you use, always moisturize when you're finished. Exfoliating your lips regularly helps your lipstick go on more smoothly and helps your lips appear younger and smoother.

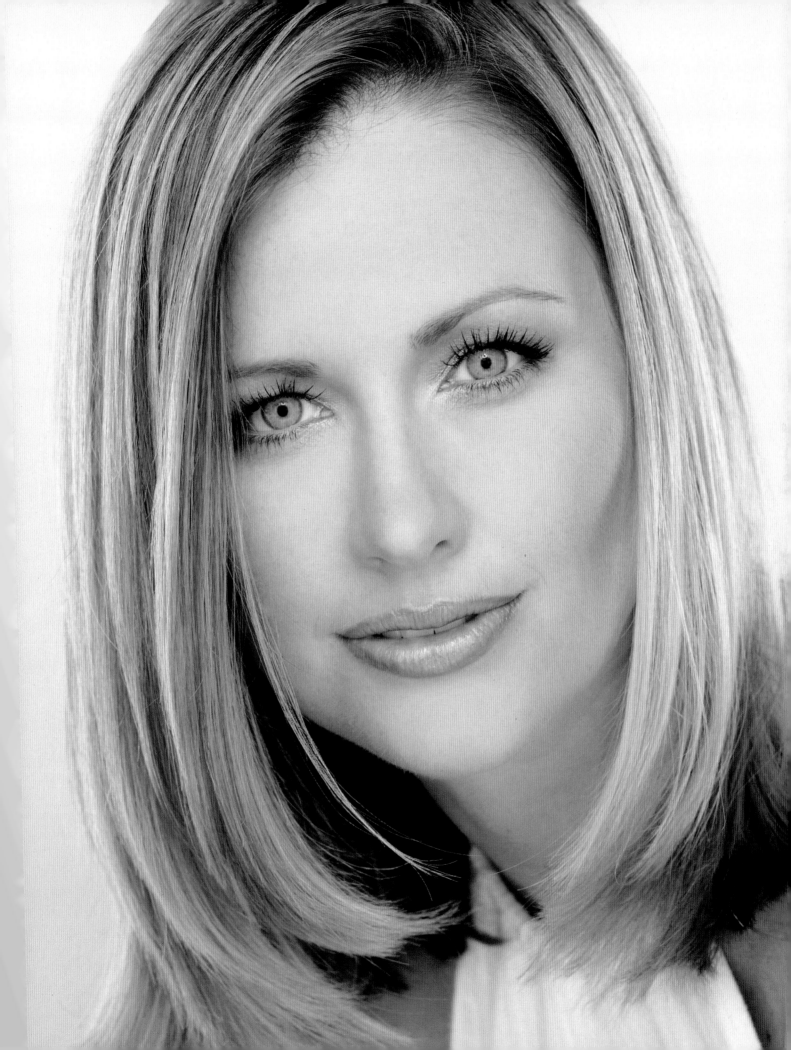

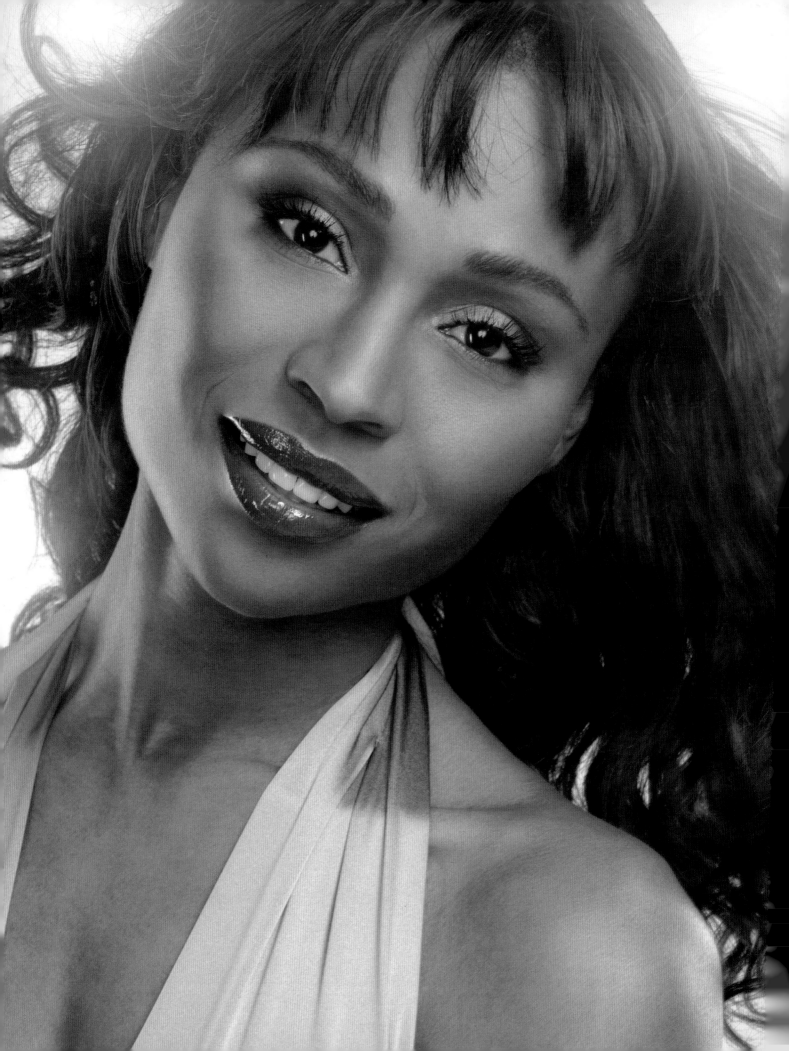

skindeep

We've all heard or even said, "My skin has a mind of its own."
And in a way that's true. Everyone has a certain skin type with its
very own characteristics. Once you know yours, it makes it easier
for you to know which foundations are right for your skin type. See
how simple it is to find your perfect match?

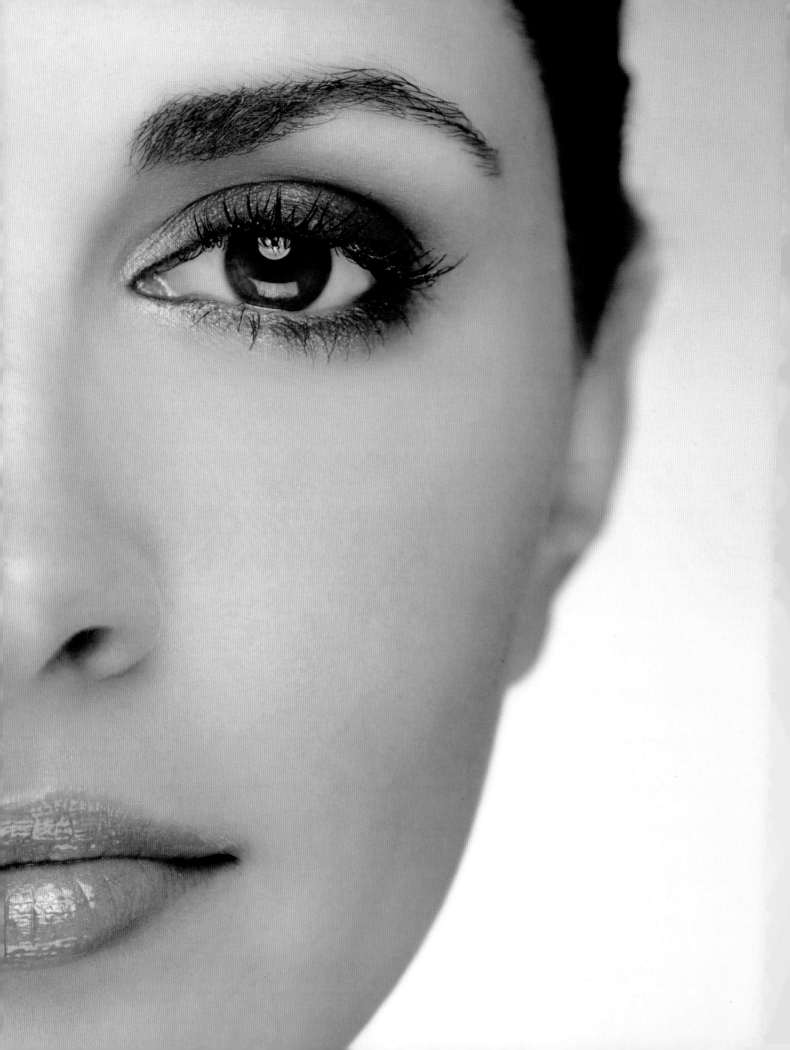

skintype	characteristics	needs	best foundation (texture)
dry	usually mature skin; lacks emollients; less elastic; rarely breaks out; feels tight after cleansing; usually small pores	moisturizing foundations; formula containing emollients and antioxidants	tinted (moisturizer); liquid (moisturizing); mousse
normal	few to no breakouts; neither too oily nor too dry; medium pores; smooth and even texture; healthy color	pH-balanced products	cream to powder; tinted (moisturizer); liquid (all types); cream; dual finish; stick; mousse
oily	prone to blackheads; large pores; gets shiny fast; breaks out often; wrinkles less; usually highly elastic	oil-free products; non-comedogenic; products enriched with oil absorbers	cream to powder; liquid (oil-free); water-based; dual finish; mousse
sensitive	burns very easily; blotchy and dry patches; more susceptible to rosacea; sensitive to many products; flushes easily; thin, delicate	hypoallergenic; fragrance-free moisturizing formulas; formulas without chemical sunscreens	liquid (water-based); mousse; tinted (moisturizer); dual finish

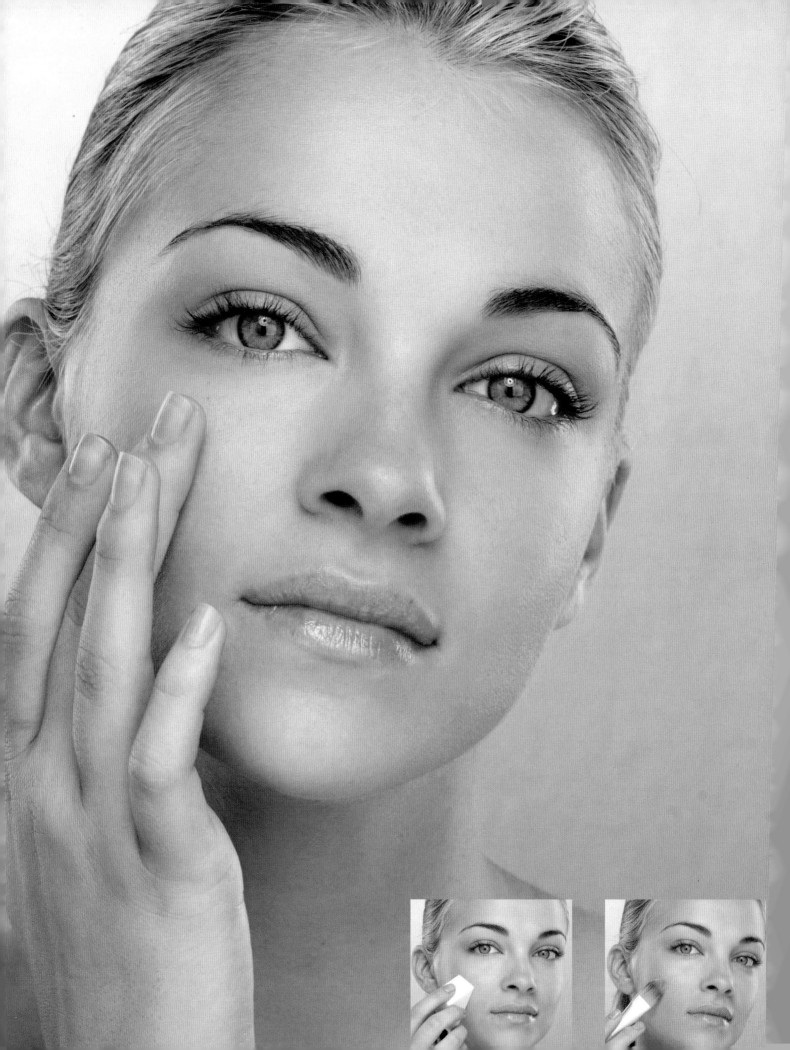

applying foundation

Selecting a foundation that's perfect for you will probably be one of your biggest makeup challenges. That's why I'm hoping the information I've given you so far can help make your selection a little easier. You'll also want to ask yourself the following questions before you set out to pick your perfect foundation:

1. What is my skin type?
2. What color undertones do I have in my skin?
3. How much coverage do I want?
4. What type of finish do I want?

The answers should help you make the correct decision. It's also important to decide what type of finish you want (see below), because some work better on certain skin types than others.

Matte is a great choice for normal/oily skin. It works best on skin with imperfections such as breakouts, scars, and discoloration. It gives you the best coverage and is perfect for oily skin because it contains no oils. However, use a light hand, because if you apply it too heavily, it can appear mask-like.

Dewy works great on dry skin because it adds moisture. It is wonderful for most skin types except oily skin, where it can increase the shine and showcase any flaws such as surface bumps or blemishes. Dewy foundation is not the best choice during summer or in high-humidity areas because it can appear too shiny or greasy instead of just dewy.

Satin works on almost all skin types, with the exception of excessively oily skin. It gives the skin a soft, smooth appearance. The finish is not as flat as matte or as shiny as dewy, but falls in between the two. Satin is the most common foundation finish.

Luminous works well on any skin type. Its light-reflecting properties help hide tiny flaws and lines by reflecting light off the surface of the face.

When applying foundation you have three basic tools at your disposal.

• A sponge is the most sanitary, because you can wash it or throw it away. Sponges also really help with the blending process.

• A brush blends well, so it gives you great even coverage. It's also great for touching up the foundation you've worn all day. It's always best to wash a sponge or a brush after every application. The cleaner the tool, the better the application.

• Don't have a brush or sponge handy? No problem, because the third tool is your fingertips. Just make sure to wash your hands after you've applied your moisturizer and treatment products and before you apply your foundation. The residue from the treatment products can compromise the integrity of your foundation and diminish the amount of coverage it provides.

BASIC

It's best to begin your application on the center of your face, dotting foundation on the cheeks and the forehead, then blending outward. Always remember to finish by blending downward to make sure all the small facial hairs lay flat. After application, blot with a tissue to absorb any oils left from the product. This will really help the staying power of your foundation. Be sure to finish with a light dusting of powder.

Tips:

The best way to achieve a natural look is to first go all over the face with a sheer foundation, then go back and dot your concealer on any small imperfections.

Foundation can also be applied to your lips. It creates a blank canvas for any reshaping you want or need to do. It's also useful as an anchor for lipstick since it helps it stay on longer.

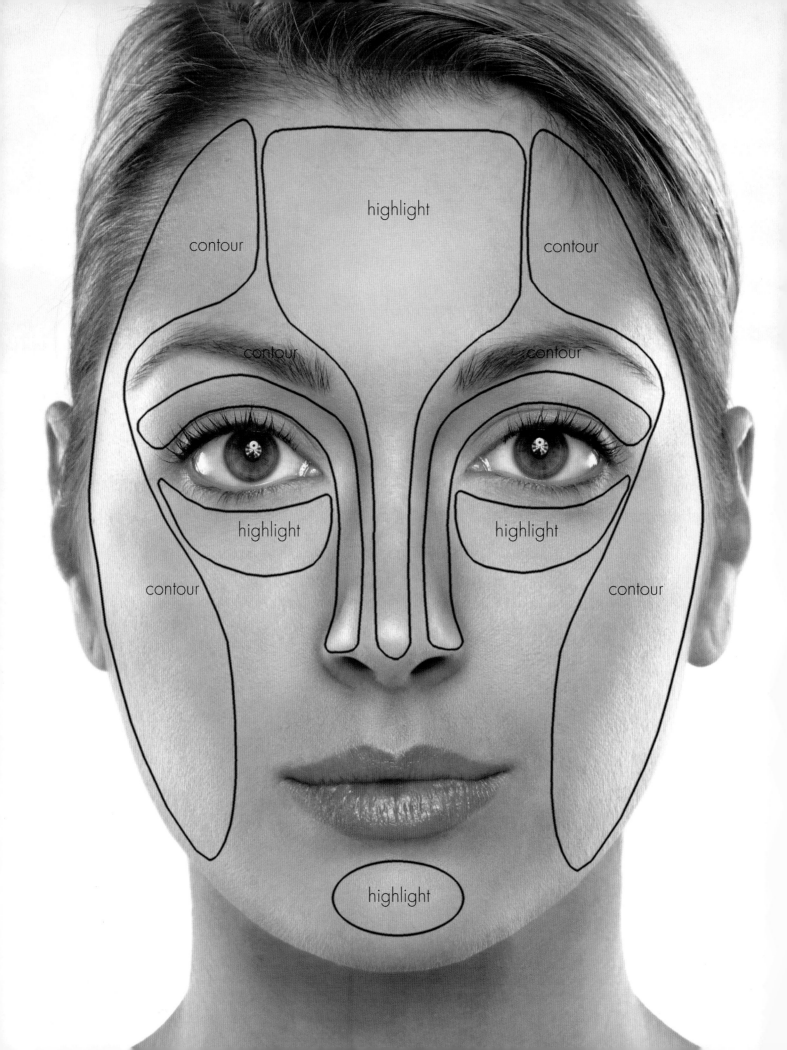

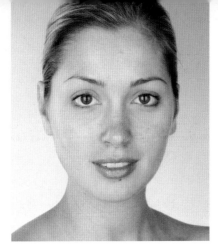

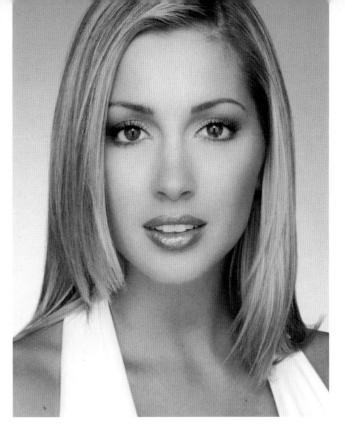

SCULPTING THE FACE

Many women with a full face want to make it appear slimmer. The most effective way to do this is to "sculpt" the face with foundation and powder. These tools can help make any face appear more oval—the face shape that is considered to be the most perfect.

No matter which products you choose, you should follow the same basic "sculpting" method. You will need to select three shades of foundation or powder in three different depth levels.

1. The first color should match your skin exactly. It is your true foundation color.

2. The second color, your highlight color, should be one level lighter than the first with the same undertone.

3. The third shade, your contour color, should be one level darker than your first with the same undertone. There should not be a dramatic difference between the three shades.

The diagram on the left will help you understand the purpose and placement of the three shades. You can also refer to the face-shape diagrams in Chapter 8, starting on page 96. Be sure to blend the three shades really well, because it is the blending process that makes the sculpting method work.

Step 1. Apply your first or true foundation color all over your face. Then visualize or trace an oval around your face. The width of the oval is your eye sockets; the height and length of your oval extends from the tip of your forehead to the tip of your chin.

Step 2. Apply your second or highlight foundation color to the high points inside the oval, including your forehead, under the eyes, on top of the cheekbones, and the tip of your chin. The features that you highlight will be what the eye will focus on first.

Step 3. Finally, use your contour or darkest shade and apply it to the areas outside the oval, including the temples, along your hairline and the sides of your cheeks. By deepening the outside areas, you are visually helping those areas recede, making your face appear more narrow and oval. If you have ivory or beige skin, you will contour your face more than highlight. On bronze and ebony skin, you will highlight your skin more than contour.

Here's an easy trick if you want to narrow the width of your nose. Highlight down the center of your nose the width that you want your nose to appear. Then place the contour shade on the sides of your nose, this will make your nose appear narrower because the eye will be drawn to the highlighted area. If your nose is a little crooked, bring a straight line down on the top of your nose with the highlighter shade, then contour along the sides. People will naturally focus on the line, making the nose appear straight.

To complete your sculpted look, you can finish with three shades of powder: one that matches your true foundation shade, one that matches your highlighter shade, and a darker or bronzing powder to match your contour shade. This will give you a beautifully sculpted, three-dimensional effect that should make any face shape appear more oval.

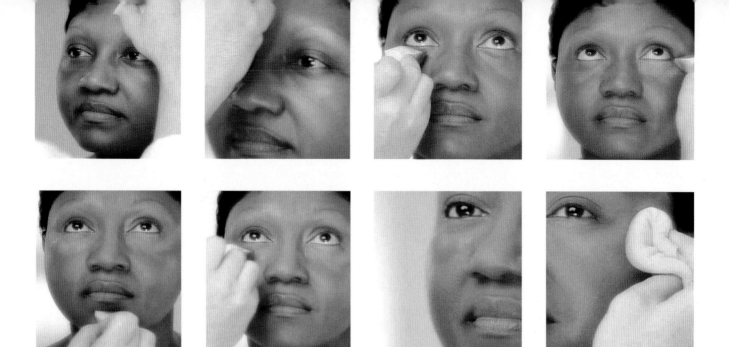

FACIAL MASKING

If your skin has a natural "mask" to it, that is, it has
a tendency to be darker around the outer edges of
the face and lighter on the interior of the face, you have
a condition called facial masking, which sometimes
occurs in women with bronze and ebony skin tones.
With a little practice, it's easy to correct facial masking
by using the following simple application techniques:

1. First, it's essential to conduct a stripe test across
the cheek and the jaw to determine the two foundation
shades you will need to create a more even look. (See
page 56 for this technique.) It takes two foundation
shades to correct your facial masking: one to brighten
the darker areas and one to deepen the lighter areas.
The goal of your stripe test is to find the two shades that,
when applied to the opposite areas of your skin, meet in
between and give you a more even skin tone.

2. Apply the lightest shade to the darker areas
and blend well.

3. Apply the darkest shade to the lighter areas
and blend well.

4. Finish with the face-sculpting technique
described on page 83, using two loose powders—
one to match your natural color and one to highlight
the "oval" on your face, including your forehead,
under the eyes, on top of the cheekbones, and the
tip of your chin.

phyllis r. sammons

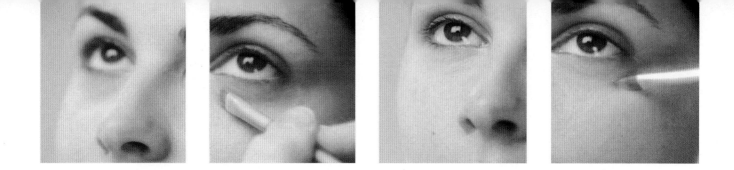

concealer

Concealer can improve your skin's appearance dramatically, but only if it's invisible. The secret to concealing everything that you do not want to see is applying concealer just to the discolored skin (learning to color within the lines, just like when you learned to color as a child). To cover under-eye discoloration (which is really blood vessels that appear blue or gray when they reflect light), you need to choose the perfect shade and texture. If you use a formula that is too moist, it can "travel," slipping into creases and fine lines, drawing attention to what you don't want people to notice. A formula that is too dry is bad for the delicate skin around the eyes and can draw attention to those same flaws. You might need to experiment to find the perfect formula for you. You should choose the same shade as your foundation, or a shade or two lighter if you have truly dark under-eye circles.

If you're using a concealer that matches your foundation exactly you may apply it either before or after your foundation. But if you're using one that is lighter, it is best to apply it first.

DARK CIRCLES

First, prepare the area underneath the eye by applying eye crème and letting it soak in for two or three minutes. Blot away any excess with a sponge or tissue. Using eye crème will help your concealer adhere, and if the skin under your eyes tends to be dry, your concealer won't "cake up" and give you an undesirable appearance. Remember, the under-eye area contains fewer oil glands than anywhere else on your body, so it needs plenty of moisture. Be generous with your eye crème, because it's next to impossible to "over-moisturize" this area. Just be sure to blot off any excess crème after a few minutes to make sure your concealer stays put.

Next, take a brush and apply concealer along the line of demarcation—where the discoloration begins on your skin. Extend the concealer up and over the discolored area with the brush. You never want to apply the concealer below the line of demarcation. If you do, you will lighten skin that is already the correct color, and you'll be back where you started—with two uneven shades of skin. Next, take your finger and, using a stippling motion, pat the concealer along the line of demarcation to blend it in. Be sure to conceal any darkness in the corners of your eyes or eyelids, if necessary.

Serious dark circles call for serious concealer. Use a shade or two lighter than your foundation and apply the concealer before your foundation. When applying your foundation, be sure to stipple or pat it on over the concealed area. You don't want to wipe away what you initially applied. Yellow concealers are a great choice for covering dark circles on ivory and beige skin. And golden-orange concealers work great for covering dark circles on bronze and ebony skin. Both concealers can counteract all shades of skin discoloration, from red to purple to brown.

Tip:

If you have mature skin, concealer and heavy powder can settle into undereye lines and wrinkles. Since you won't want to accentuate them with too much powder, use your fingertip to dab on just the tiniest trace

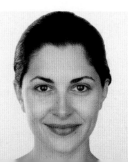

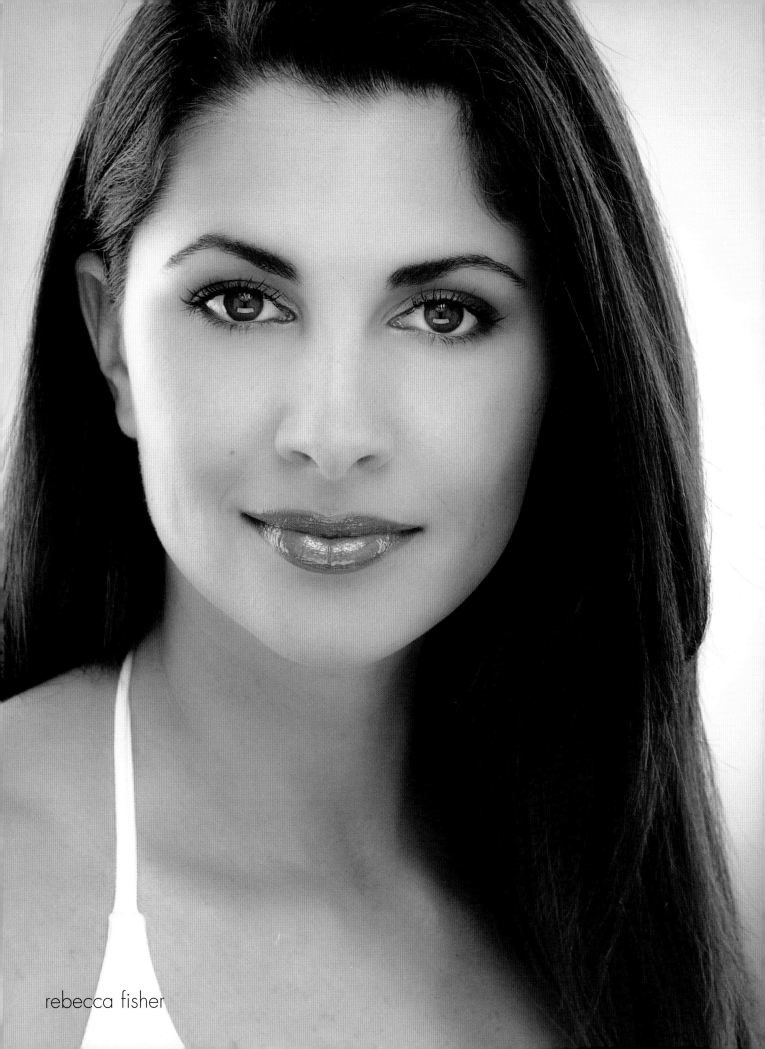

rebecca fisher

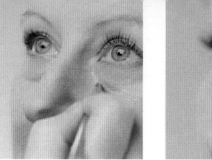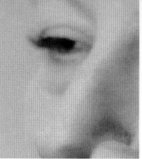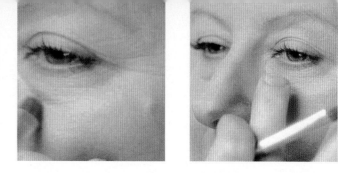

UNDER-EYE PUFFINESS

As painful as it is to admit this, you cannot improve the appearance of under-eye puffiness by swiping a light concealer under the eye area. By now we know that anything we highlight on the face makes it stand out more. Our goal is to disguise the puffy area—not make it more prominent.

You can outsmart the puffy area by highlighting the area just underneath it. Because our faces are lit from above, the puffy area creates a shadow on the face. By highlighting the shadowy area, you will bring it out and make the puffiness recede. Because most people look directly at you and not from above, your puffiness will appear even with the rest of your skin. Voilà—you're flawless!

To apply, take a fine-tipped brush and apply a light-colored concealer just underneath the puffy area. Then lightly blend it with your finger, using a stippling motion. If you have dark circles as well as puffiness, which many women do, you'll want to use this three-step application:

1. Apply concealer to your dark circles first.
2. Next, apply your foundation to the rest of your face.
3. Finally, highlight underneath the puffiness with your concealer. This is one time that you will apply a lighter concealer after your foundation and not completely blend it away. Be sure to use a stippling motion to blend well.

Tips:

Using a concealer that's too light will only draw attention to what you're trying to cover.

Concealer can be made sheerer by mixing it with a little eye crème.

You can test coverage by applying a little concealer to a vein on the inside of your wrist.

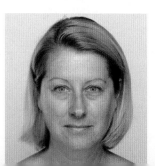

madeleine zeisler

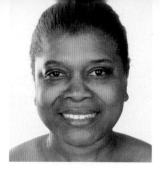

skin imperfections

Let's face it: Very few women have perfectly flawless skin. Everything from sun damage to genetics can affect the surface of your complexion. Fortunately, there are several different concealers with different textures to help you tackle your problem areas and help your skin look its best.

BLEMISHES

To minimize facial blemishes, you'll want to use a dry-textured concealer so it will cling better to the blemish and not irritate the skin. Apply your foundation first and make sure to choose a concealer that matches your skin exactly. (A light concealer will only make the blemish seem larger.) Using a brush, apply the concealer directly to the blemish. Then take your finger and, using a stippling motion, blend the edges around the blemish into the skin.

BROKEN CAPILLARIES OR VEINS

Here, as always, it's important to apply concealer only to the areas of discoloration. You can take a brush and actually draw a line of concealer on top of the broken capillary or vein. Then stipple out the edges to blend.

ROSACEA

To counteract the redness of rosacea, you should use a yellow-based concealer and apply it only to the reddened areas of your face. Then stipple the outer edges with your fingertips and gently blend into skin. Finish by stippling foundation over the area so it will match your skin tone exactly.

HYPERPIGMENTATION OR MELASMA

Age spots or brown spots can be caused by too much sun or by a shift in hormones during pregnancy. To correct them, you'll want to apply concealer only to the areas that are discolored. Otherwise, if you extend the

concealer past the line of demarcation, you will lighten skin that is already the correct color. After applying, you'll want to stipple the edges to blend the concealer. Finish by stippling foundation over the area so it will match your skin tone exactly. Women with ivory and beige skin tones should use an intense yellow concealer. If you have bronze or ebony skin tones, you should use a golden-orange concealer.

SCARS

A scar is a raised area of skin that has no pores, which makes it difficult to conceal because pores are what makeup clings to. To conceal a scar, apply a drier-textured concealer with a brush directly onto the scar. Then stipple the edges to blend it in. If you don't have a dry concealer for scars, try this treatment: Apply moisturizer to the scarred area, followed by a bit of loose powder. The moisturizer gives the powder something to cling to. Then take a brush and apply concealer right onto the scar. The concealer and the powder mix together to form a drier texture that will stick.

Remember that concealers are very different from foundations. They are drier, more heavily pigmented, and they "grab" powder differently. If there is an area that you have heavily concealed it is best to use a lighter shade of powder on this area. If you use the same shade of powder as on the rest of your face, the concealed area may appear darker.

For acne scars, which create texture variation, the best way to make the skin look perfectly flawless is to keep it as matte as possible. Loose powder is your best friend, because it will do just that for you. The last thing you will want to do is to try to fill in the "valleys" by applying too much foundation and concealer.

ann brown

powder

Powder is a makeup must. It sets your foundation, polishes your look, and adds a smooth, velvety softness to the skin. Because loose powder contains more oil absorbers, I prefer to use it to set the foundation, then use pressed powder for touch-ups throughout the day. There are several ways to apply both types of powder:

• A sponge works well for tight areas and is great for "spot" powdering.

• A brush is the easiest and most commonly used tool. It is great for blending, but you must be careful not to over-blend and brush off what you apply. For best results, apply a little bit of powder at a time with a brush, instead of applying it all at once, to ensure smooth, even coverage.

• A powder puff offers the best coverage and is my favorite way to apply powder. Press a puff or sponge into the powder and then "roll" it onto the skin. Pushing it into the skin makes your foundation and powder appear as one with your skin and looks far more natural. To finish, lightly sweep the face with a brush using gentle downward strokes to remove any excess powder.

• A fingertip works well for a light powder application. It's a great way to powder underneath the eyes, especially for mature women. Just dip your finger in loose powder. Rub your finger in the palm of your hand to brush off the excess, then trace your finger over the area underneath the eyes to set your concealer and help minimize fine lines.

Tips:

Yellow-based shades look healthier and more natural.

To get that perfect shade of concealer, try mixing it with a little of your foundation.

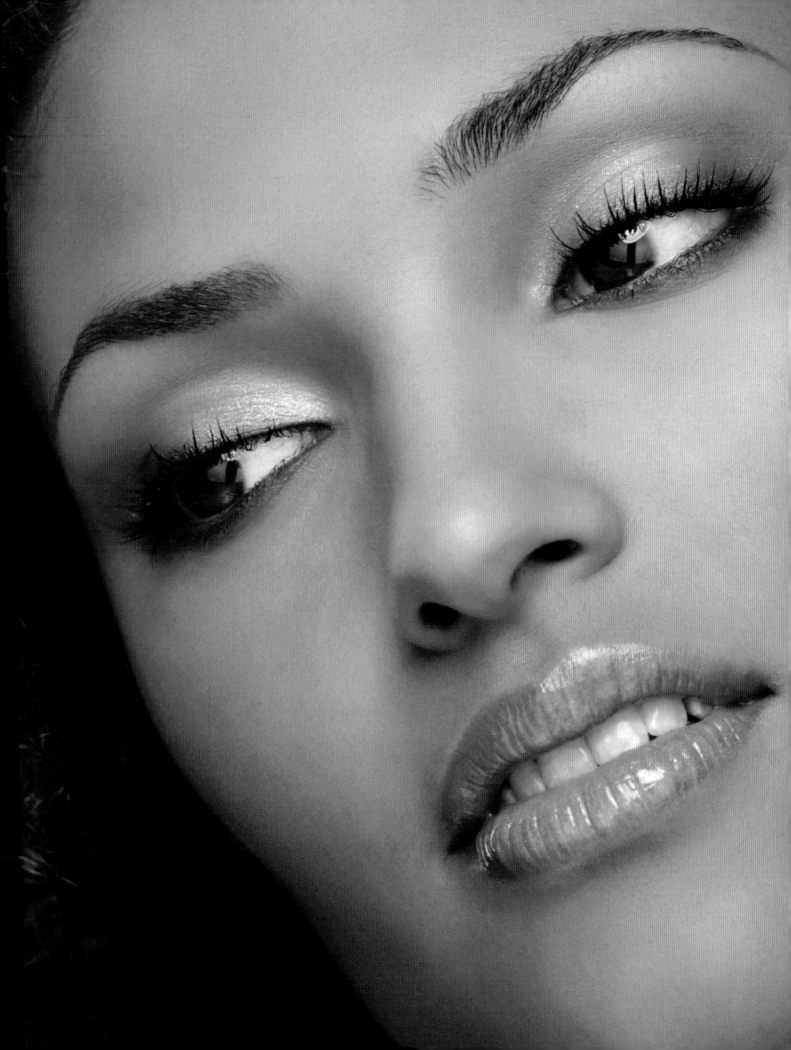

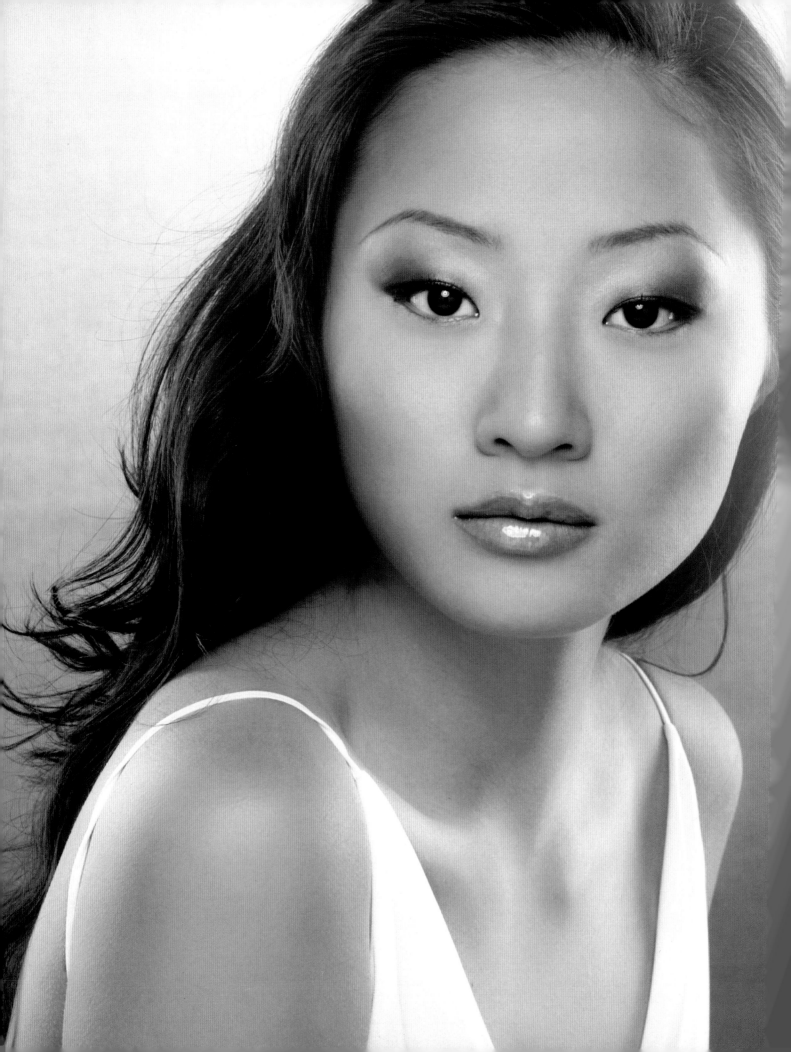

faceshape

8

Everything about your face is unique, including its shape. So why would you want to put on your makeup the same way as everyone else? Here, I'll show you the different face shapes and teach you how to apply your makeup to enhance the real you.

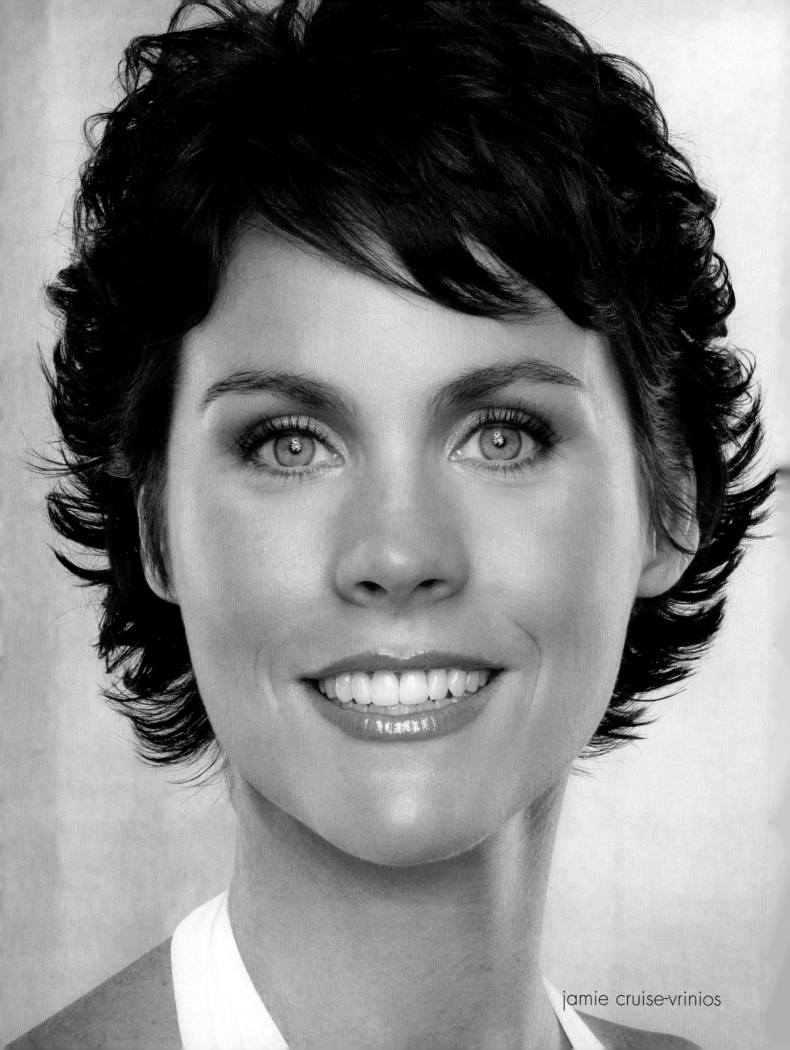

jamie cruise-vrinios

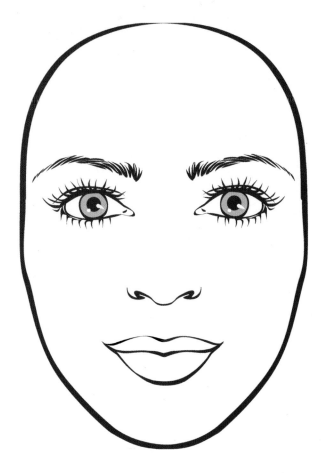

oval face

An oval-shaped face is considered by most to be the perfect facial shape because of its beautiful symmetry. It is usually broader at the cheeks, tapering in slightly at both the forehead and the chin. Because of its symmetry, you do not need to contour and highlight your face. You can experiment and play all you want. An oval face can support most makeup trends—so have fun!

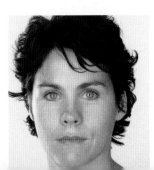

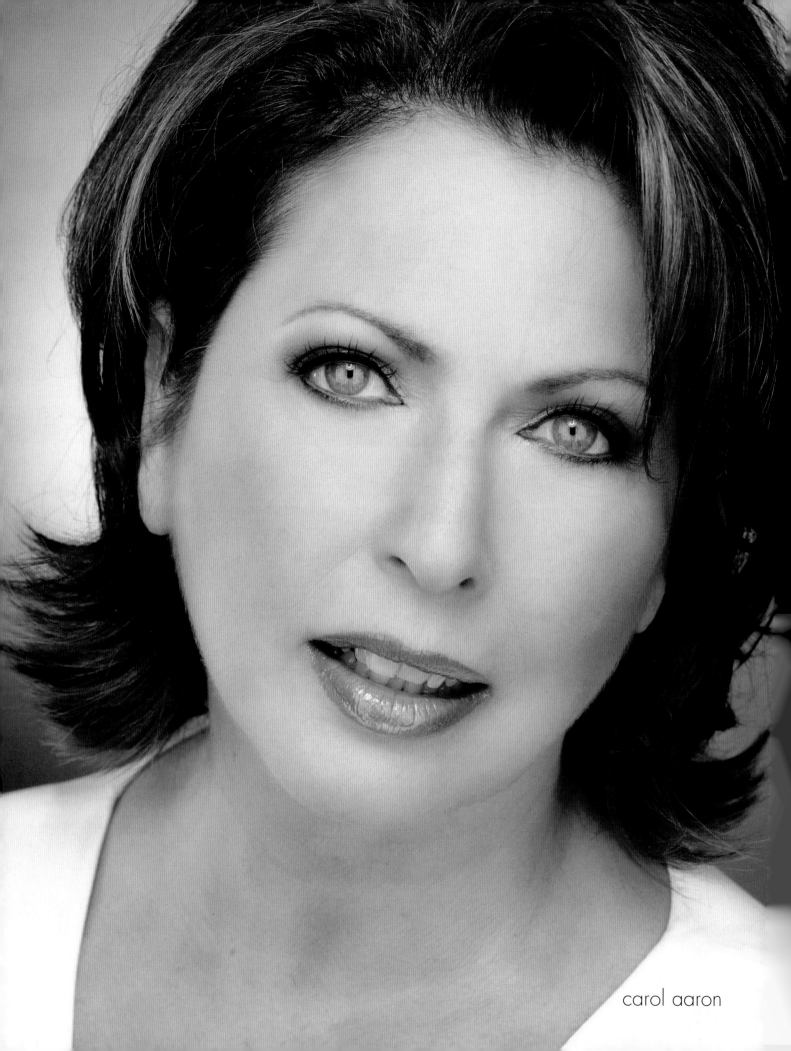

carol aaron

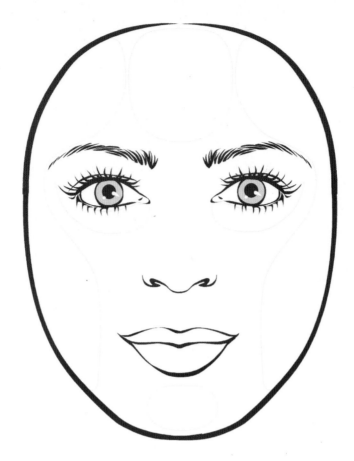

round face

A round-shaped face is fuller and generally holds its youthful appearance longer than the other face shapes. It's shorter, fairly wide, with full cheeks and a rounded chin.

IF YOU HAVE A ROUND-SHAPED FACE:

• Highlight your forehead, underneath the eyes just on top of the cheekbones, and the center of your chin to draw attention to the center of your face.

• Contour your temples, cheeks, and jawline with a bronzer or a product that is one or two levels darker than your skin tone to create the illusion of an oval.

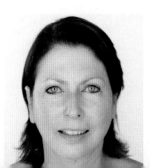

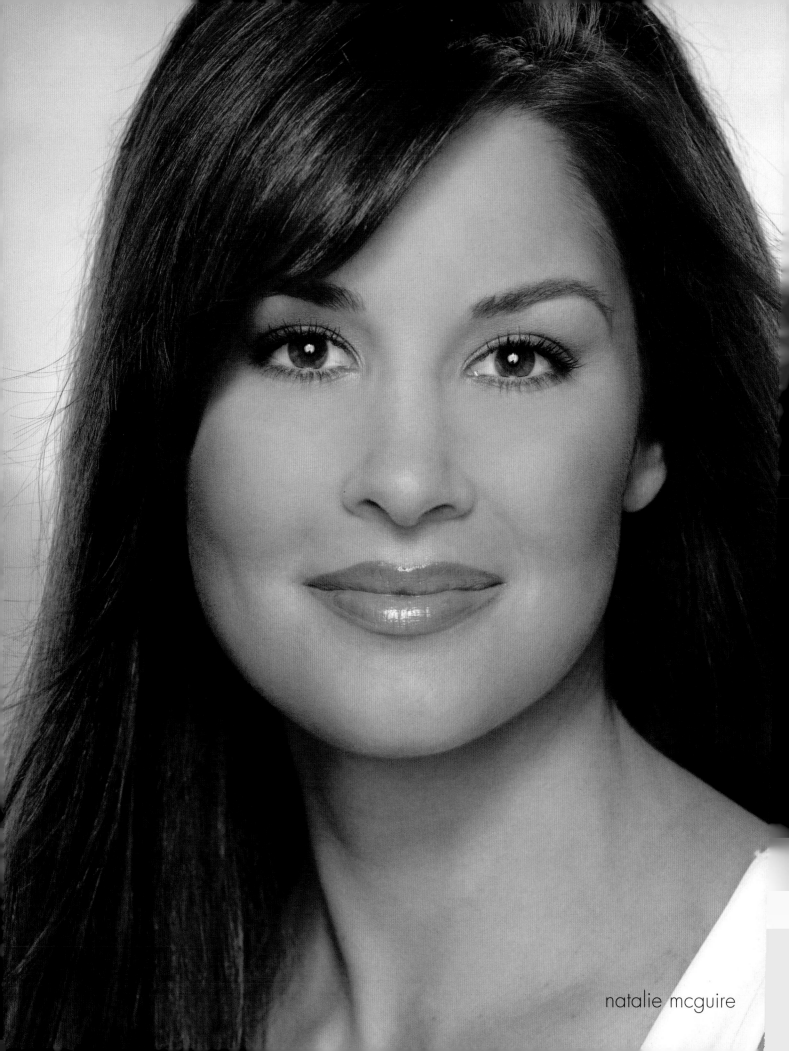

natalie mcguire

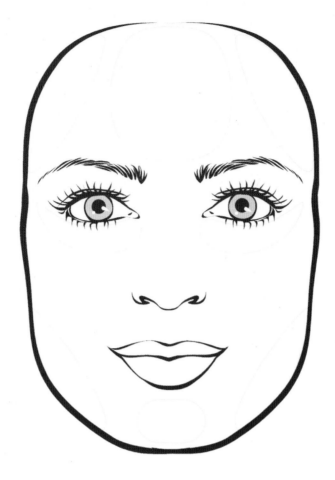

square face

A square-shaped face is the same width at the forehead, the cheeks, and the jaw.

IF YOU HAVE A SQUARE-SHAPED FACE:

• Highlight down the center of your forehead, underneath the eyes just on top of the cheekbones, and the tip of your chin to draw attention to the middle of your face.

• Contour your hairline at the two corners by your temples and the jaw at the two corners.

• Apply blush on the apples of your cheeks to help draw attention away from the corners of the square and help widen the area and make it appear more oval.

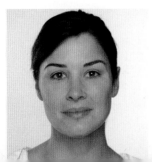

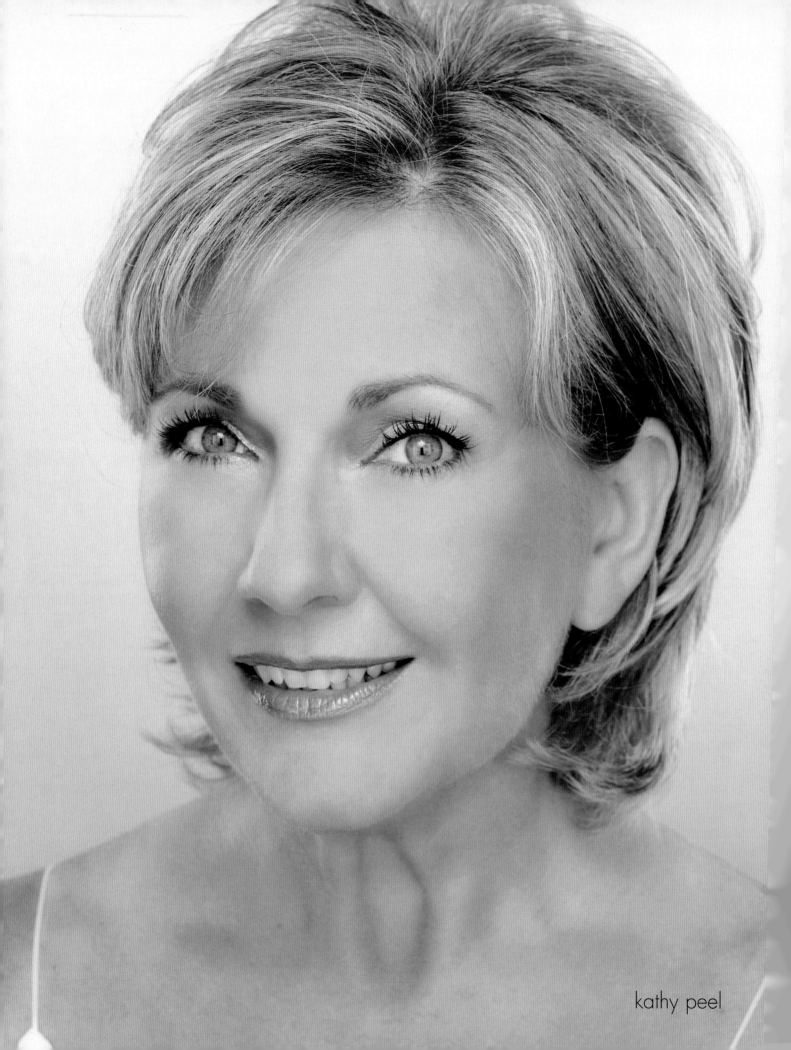

kathy peel

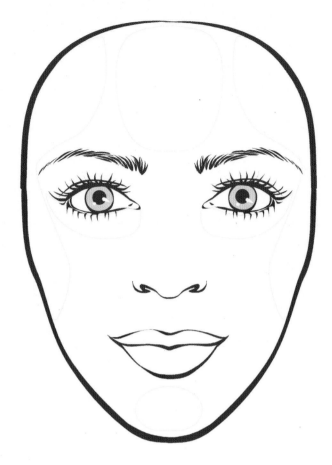

heart-shaped face

The heart-shaped face is wide at the forehead and curves down to a pointed or narrow chin, like an inverted triangle.

IF YOU HAVE A HEART-SHAPED FACE:

• Highlight the chin to help broaden it. Highlight the forehead and underneath the eyes just on top of the cheekbones to draw attention to the center of your face.

• Contour the temples and cheeks to diminish the width of this portion of your face.

Tip:

Pressed powder works well for sculpting the face because it's low in pigment and blends easily. Or, if you like, you could use a bronzer; just be sure to blend really well.

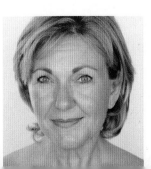

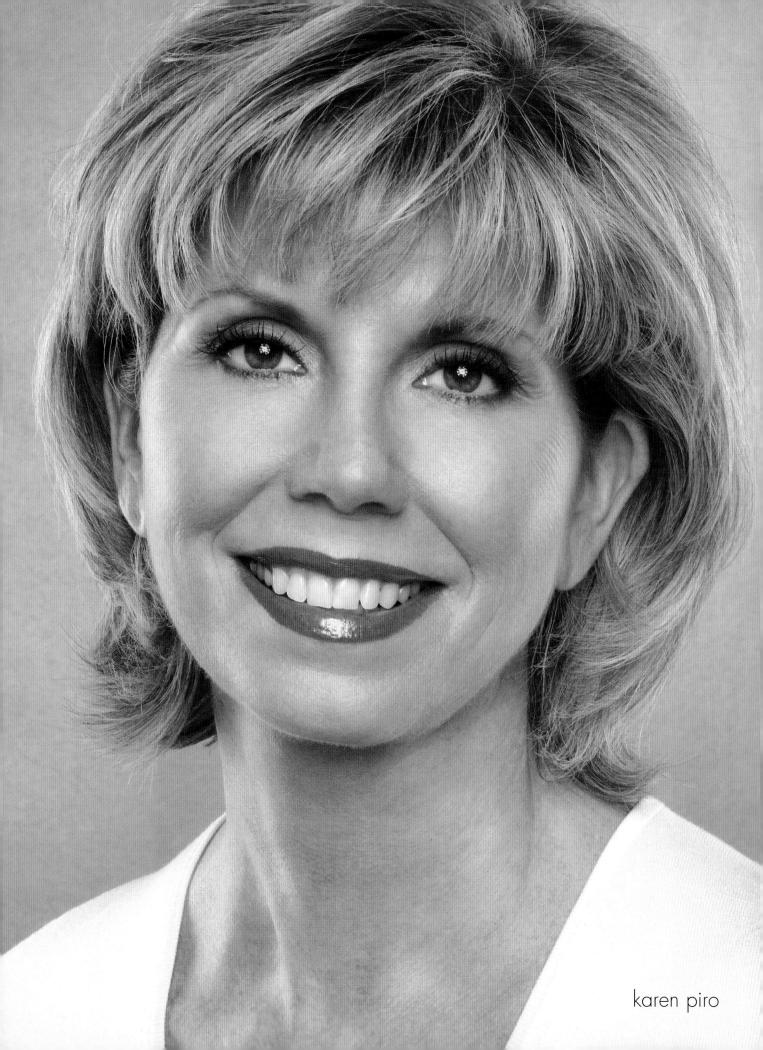

karen piro

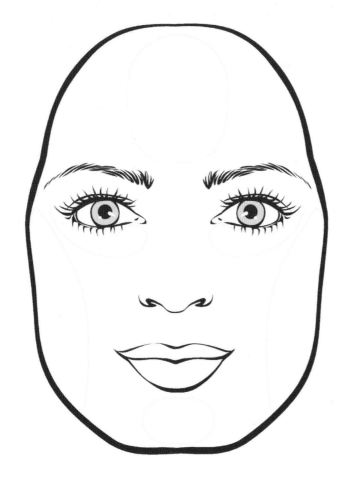

pear-shaped face

The pear-shaped face is narrow at the temples and forehead and wider at the cheeks and jawline.

IF YOU HAVE A PEAR-SHAPED FACE:

• Highlight your forehead to create the illusion of width, and highlight underneath the eyes on top of the cheekbones and the tip of your chin.

• Contour the jawline and the cheeks to minimize their width.

Tip:

Remember that the proper hairstyle can go a long way in balancing any face shape. In this case, bangs and hair brushed over the temples add fullness to the upper half of the face.

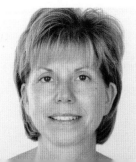

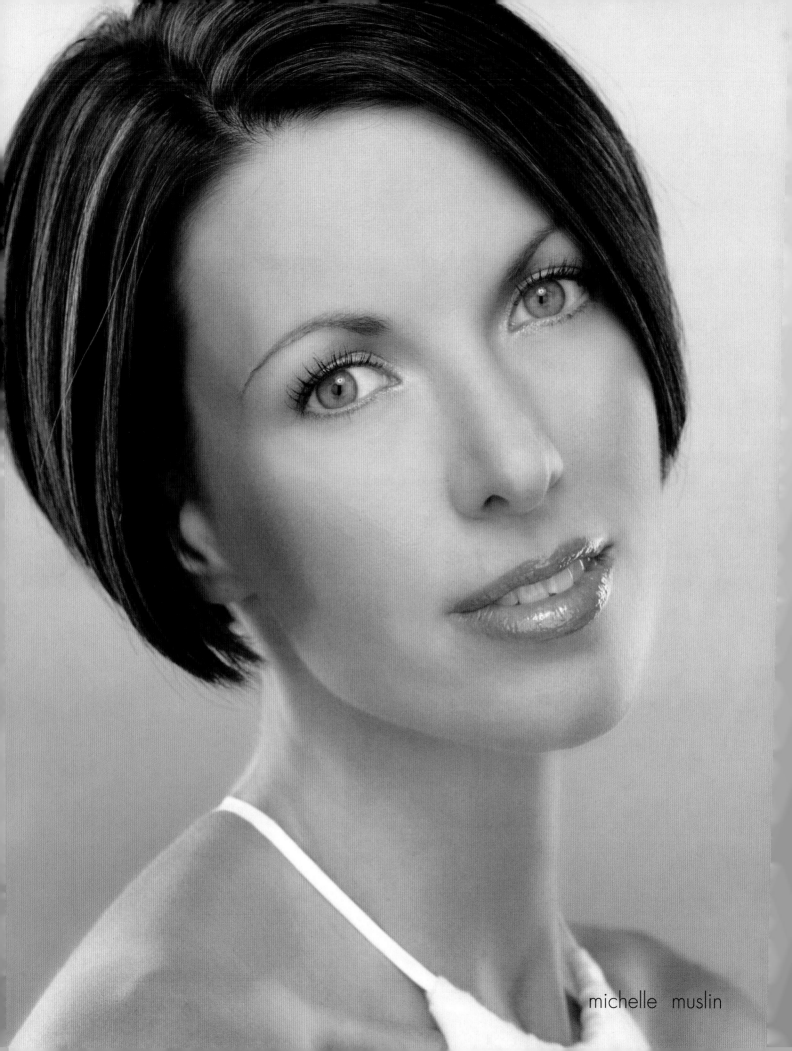
michelle muslin

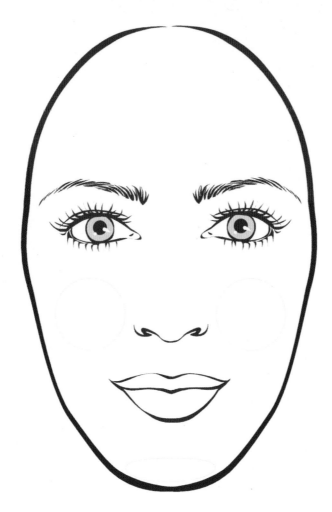

long face

The long face has high cheekbones, a high, deep forehead, and a strong, sharp, chiseled jawline.

IF YOU HAVE A LONG FACE:

• Never highlight or contour your face. This will only make your face appear even longer.

• Brush a bit of bronzer across your chin to help shorten its length.

• Be generous with your blush and place a lot of color on the apples of your cheeks. This will help widen and shorten your face.

• Bangs can help shorten the length of your face as well.

Tip:

When applying your blush, start closer in on the apples of the cheeks and brush outward across the face.

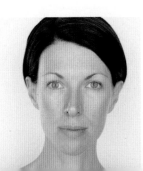

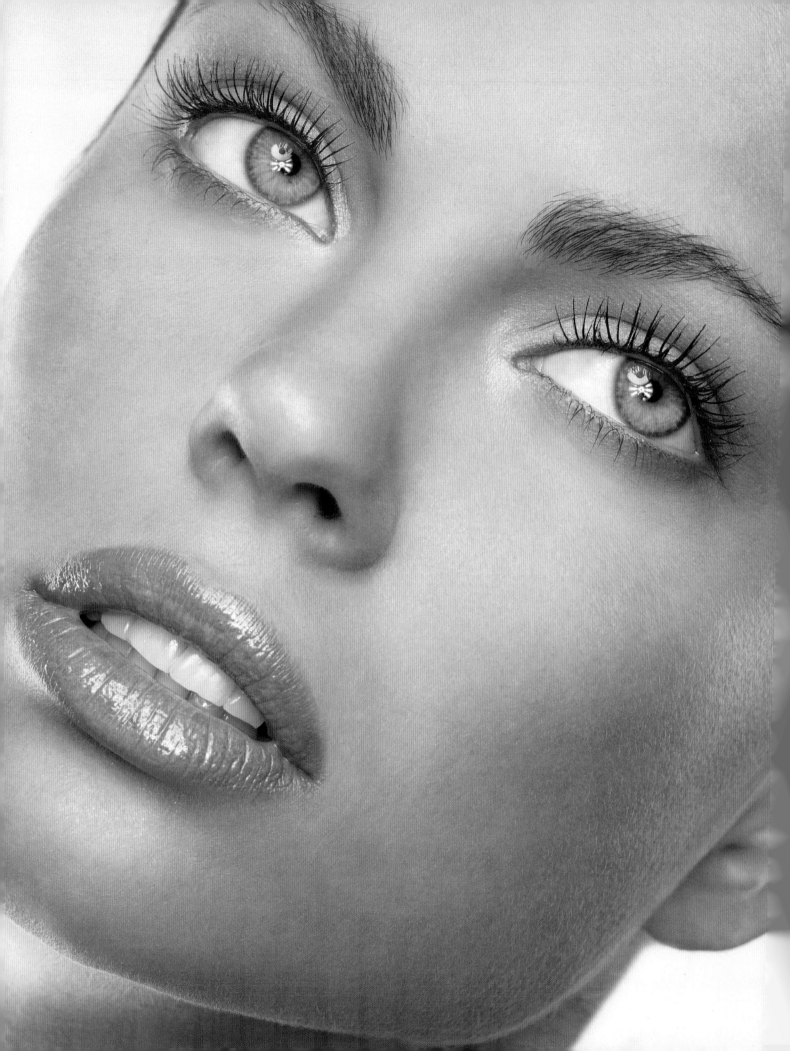

eye**shape**

9

To master the art of eye color application, it's helpful to understand how the shape and spacing of your eyes can determine the placement of color and the effect it creates. Together, we'll look at a variety of different eye shapes and application techniques developed to maximize the individuality and beauty of each. Prepare to see the world of eye color application in a whole new way!

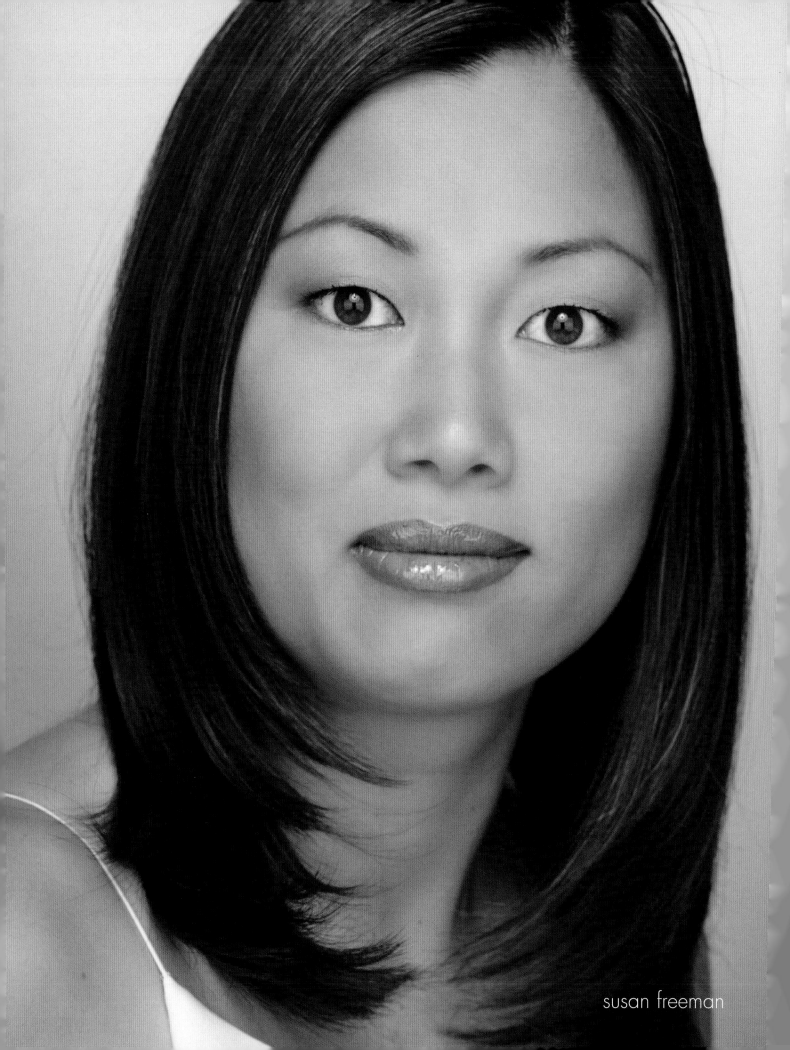

susan freeman

hooded eyes

Hooded eyes are sometimes called "bedroom eyes" because the lids tend to look partly closed. Applied correctly, eye color can help hooded eyes appear more open by minimizing the eyelid. Our goal is to make the fleshy lid area "push away" or recede, and help your eyes become more prominent than the eyelids.

- Never use a dark eyeshadow over the entire lid, because it makes it appear heavier and will close in your eyes.
- Don't be tempted to highlight the browbone too much, because doing so can accentuate the hooded appearance of the eyelid.

Tip:

The eyebrow shape is very important here, because attention can be diverted from the hooded eyelid with a beautifully shaped eyebrow.

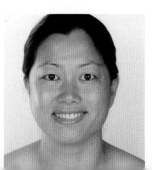

APPLICATION:

1. Highlight shade: Apply to browbone and along the upper lash line.

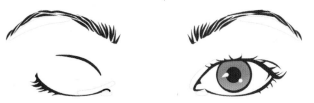

2. Midtone shade: Start at the base of your upper lash line and bring the color up and over the entire hooded area. This helps the lid recede. Make sure to blend the areas where the midtone color meets the highlight color.

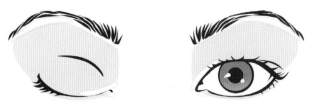

3. Contour shade: Start at the base of the lash line and bring the color up and over the hooded area. For this eye shape, you need to bring your contour color in a little farther and up a little higher than on other eye shapes. This will help the hooded area recede. Next, sweep the contour color underneath the lower lashes to define the lower lashline. You don't want to miss this step! Hooded eyes really benefit from a well-defined upper and lower lash line.

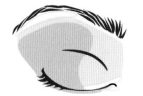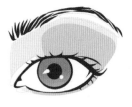

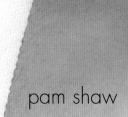
pam shaw

wide-set eyes

If the spacing between your eyes is wider than the width of one eye, your eyes are considered wide-set. Your goal is to create the illusion that they are set closer together.

• In this case, you need to darken the inside hollows of your eye next to the bridge of your nose more than for any other eye shape. Deepening the color helps this area appear to recede and makes your eyes look closer together.

• Begin all dark-color application slightly in from the outer corners and blend your shadow in and up instead of outward, because an outward blending will "pull" the eyes wider apart, and your goal is to "pull" them closer together.

APPLICATION:

1. Highlight shade: Apply to browbone and lid.

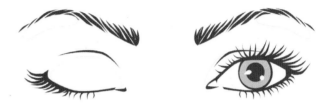

2. Midtone shade: Starting from the outer corner of the crease, bring the color towards the inside corner of your eye. Be sure to apply a few more layers to the inside corners to deepen the color and help visually push the eyes closer together.

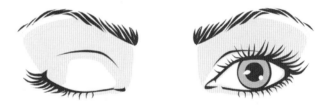

3. Contour shade: Starting slightly in from the outer corner, brush it across the upper lash line and up into the crease of your eye. Also sweep it underneath the lower lash line, being careful not to extend the color beyond the outer edge of the eye.

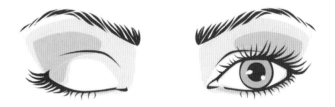

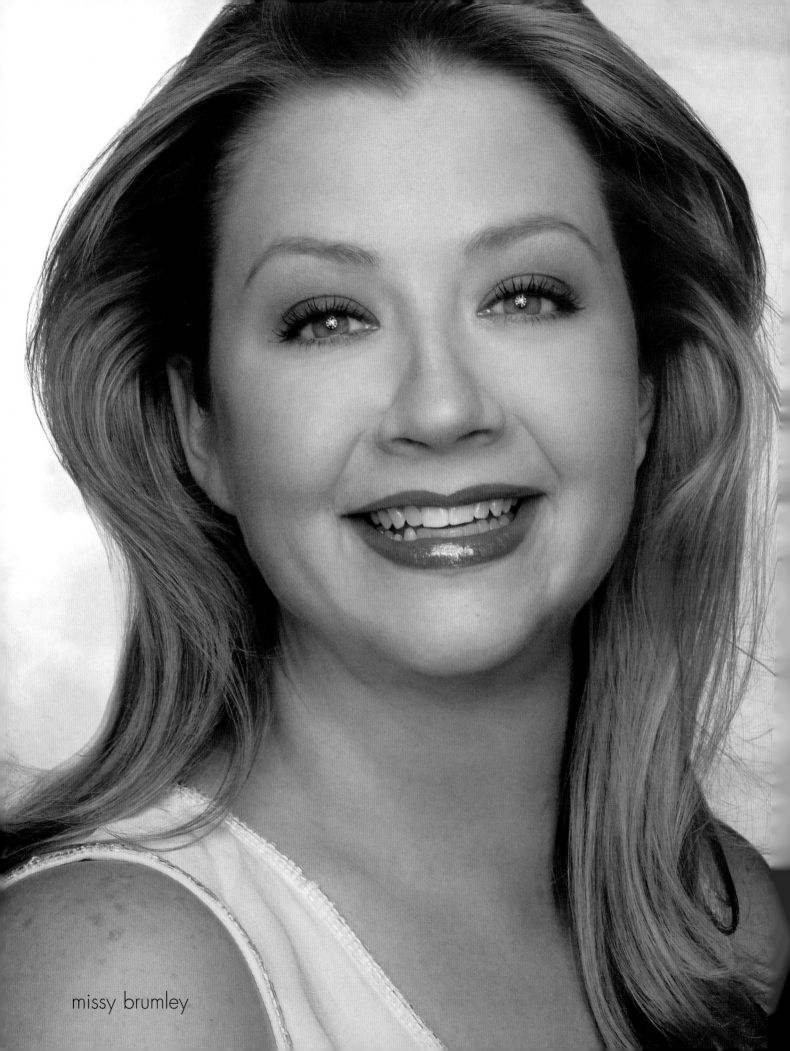
missy brumley

prominent eyes

If your eyelids and eyes are very full and tend to extend from the face, you have prominent eyes. The goal here is to visually "push" the eye away from us and help it appear to recede more gently into the face. We do this by creating a light-to-dark effect with the three eyeshadows, with the darkest shade applied closest to the lash line and fading as you go toward the brow.

• Never highlight the eyelid, or you will make the eye appear even more prominent.

• A deeper or contour shade across the lid helps to minimize it and makes it appear to recede.

APPLICATION:

1. Highlight shade: Apply to browbone only.

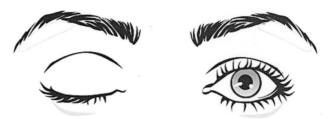

2. Midtone shade: Start at the base of your upper lash line and bring the color up and over your entire lid, all the way up to your browbone.

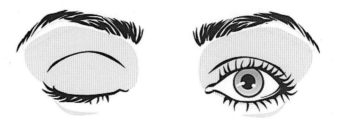

3. Contour shade: Again, start at the base of your lash line, and bring the color all the way across the lid and up into the crease. Then sweep the contour color underneath the lower lash line as well.

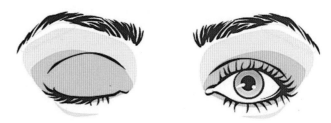

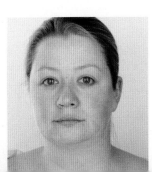

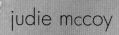
judie mccoy

deep-set eyes

Deep-set eyes are eyes that are set deep into the sockets. The browbone also extends out farther than with any other eye shape. The goal with deep-set eyes is to bring them out and make them more noticeable.

• A dark eyelid does not work with this eye shape. You want to highlight deep-set eyes as much as possible to help bring them out.

• A dark crease is also unnecessary for this eye shape. Nature has provided its own, so there's no need to emphasize it.

• There is no need to highlight the browbone, since it is already prominent.

• If you wear eyeliner with this eye shape, keep it very close to the lash line and very thin. A thick eyeliner will work against you when you're trying to bring the eye out, especially on the upper lid.

Tips:

Never darken your lid, because it can close in your eyes and make them appear smaller.

For drama, I always use a brighter (not necessarily a darker) color of shadow.

APPLICATION:

1. Highlight shade: Apply to the eyelid and in the crease.

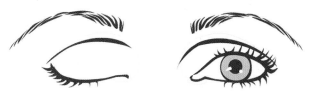

2. Midtone shade: Bring the color up above the crease and sweep it across the browbone to help visually "push" the browbone away from us.

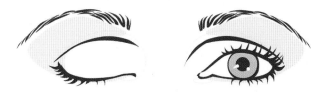

3. Contour shade: Apply to the outer corner of the upper lash line, then up onto the corner of the browbone to help "push" the area away, or recede. Sweep the contour shade underneath the lower lash line for definition.

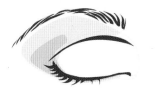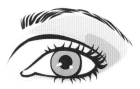

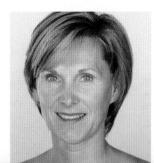

taylor moore

close-set eyes

The average space between a pair of eyes is approximately the width of one eye. If your eyes are spaced any closer, you have close-set eyes. Your goal is to create the illusion of eyes that are farther apart.

• Keep the inside corners and areas closest to the nose as light as possible to help visually "push" the eyes apart.

• Make sure to concentrate the darker shades on the outer corners of this eye shape.

APPLICATION:

1. Highlight shade: Apply to lid and browbone. Also apply to the inside corner at the bottom lashline.

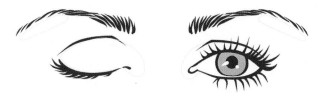

2. Midtone shade: Starting at the outer corner of the crease, bring the color in toward the inside corner to the brow but not all the way over to your nose.

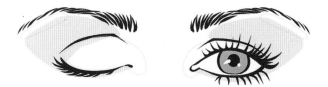

3. Contour shade: Sweep it across the base of the upper lash line and up into the outer area of the crease. Sweep it underneath the lower lash line for definition, except for the inside corners. Apply your highlight shade to the inside corners of the eye to help your eyes appear farther apart.

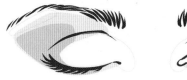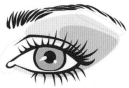

Tip:

To open up your eyes and create the illusion of larger eyes, you can apply white or beige eyeliner around the inside "wet tissue" of the eyes (the inside rim).

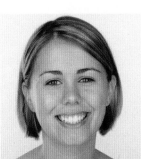

lisa madson

droopy eyes

Droopy eyes slope downward at the outer corners. They are sometimes referred to as "sad puppy-dog eyes." Your goal is to make the outer corners appear as if they turn up rather than down.

• You can do this best by creating an "open-ended" eye, which means you do not extend your colors to the outer corner of the eye where it begins to turn down. By leaving it natural, you actually create a visual "lift" to the eye.

• When applying mascara, be sure to concentrate on the middle to inside lashes. Defined lashes on the outer corner of the eye will only accentuate the droopiness.

• Make sure your eyebrows curve gently outward—never in an exaggerated downward arch.

APPLICATION:

1. Highlight shade: Apply to browbone and lid.

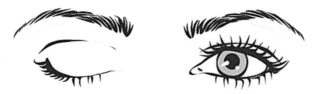

2. Midtone shade: Starting slightly in from the outside corner, bring the color across the crease into the inside corner of the crease.

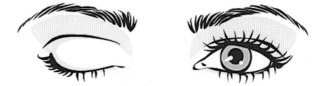

3. Contour shade: Starting just slightly in from the outside corner, bring your color up and into the crease. Next, sweep contour color along the lower lash line, making sure once again to start slightly in from the outside corner.

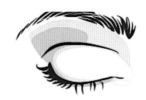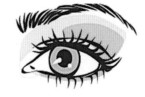

Tip:

If you want to wear color at the lower lash line, begin your application about an eighth of an inch in from the outermost corner.

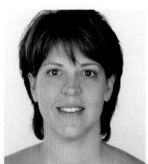

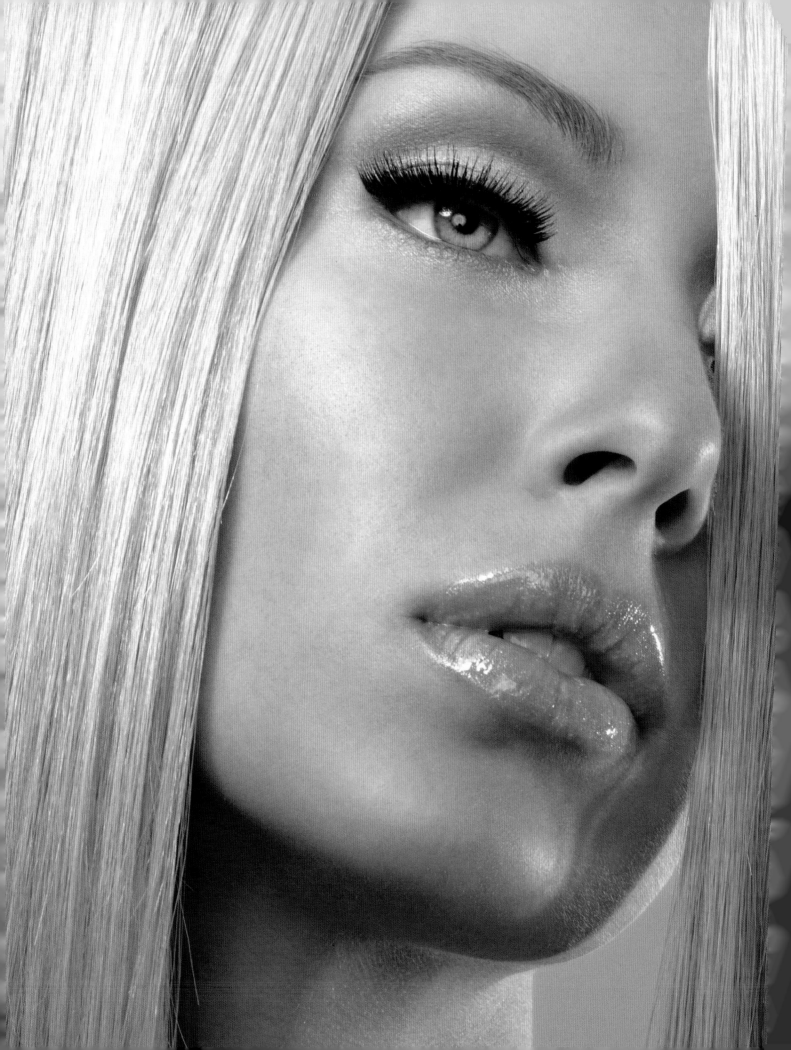

part three putting it all together

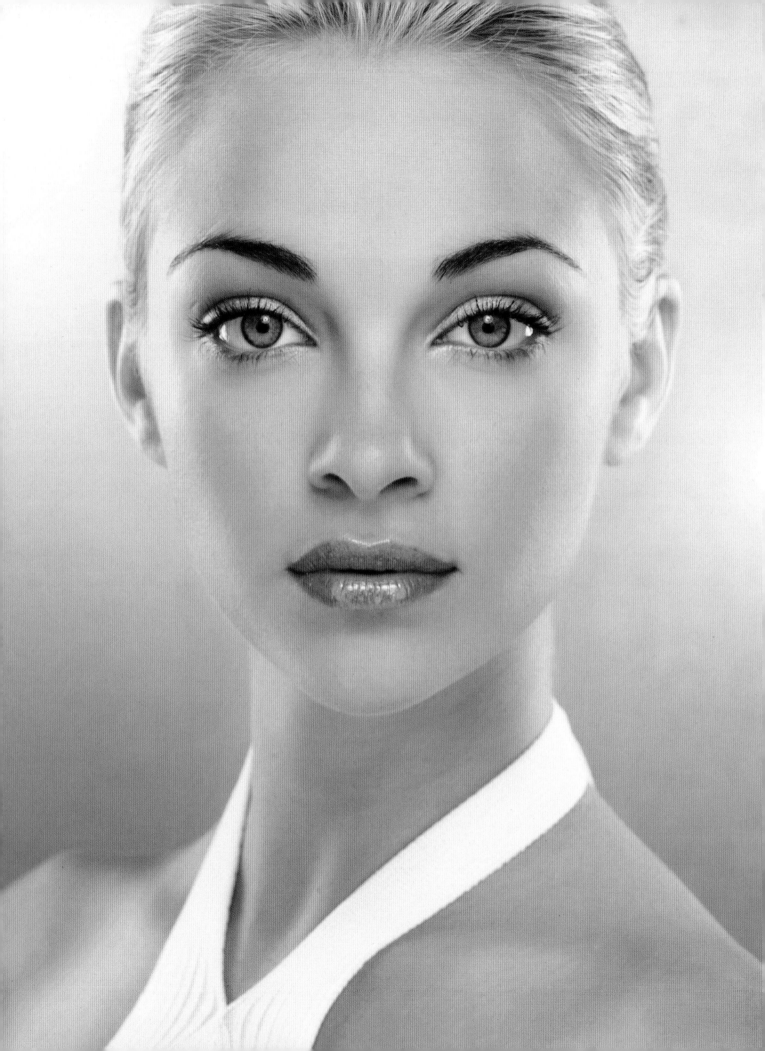

basicapplication

Girls just want to have fun—especially when it comes to makeup. So get ready to play with color! In this chapter, we'll paint on the perfect eye look, learn the tricks of applying blush and bronzers, make lips speak volumes with luscious color, and even experiment with false eyelashes. Get ready to reveal the real you!

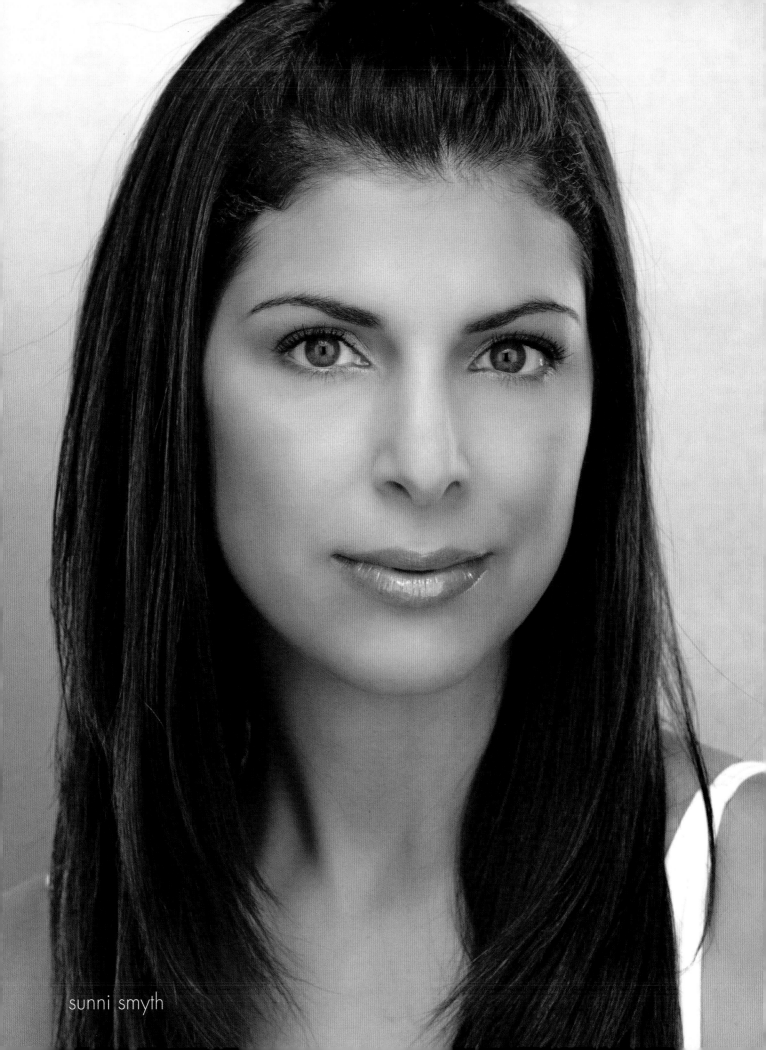
sunni smyth

brows

When selecting a brow color, choose one that is either your natural color or one shade lighter. Be careful not to confuse brow pencils and powders with eye pencils and shadows—they are not the same.

Brow pencils are duller in color, usually with no sheen, and have a somewhat waxier texture than eyeliner pencils do. Eyebrow powder is duller and more matte than eyeshadow.

When using a brow pencil, apply short, feathery, hairlike strokes angled in the same direction as the hairs' growth. Never draw on a solid, hard-looking line. Short feather-like strokes are meant to imitate short brow hairs. I like to go over the area again, using a small angled brush, following the same stroke pattern. It blends the pencil in a little better and helps it appear more natural.

You can also achieve a very natural brow by using brow powder. Apply it with a small, stiff, angled brush in short, feathery strokes, while following the natural hair growth pattern.

For those with scars or brows that are just not there, you may need the coverage of a crème brow color, which gives the most coverage. Simply apply it with a stiff, angled brush using short feathery strokes. It's always best to follow crème with a brow powder to set it and help it last all day.

Whichever method you prefer, when grooming your brows, always finish by using a brow brush to brush upward and outward. If you like, you can end with a brow gel. It acts like hairspray for the brows. To review how to create the best shape for your brows, turn to page 72.

Tips:

Sharpen your pencil each time you use it. The sharper the pencil, the better the application.

You can use eyebrow pencil or eyebrow powder separately, or you can combine them. If you combine them, you'll increase their wearing time.

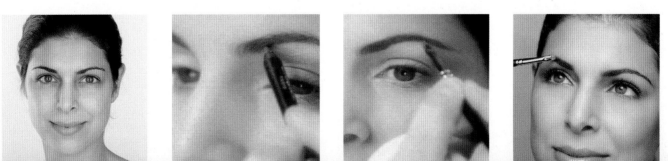

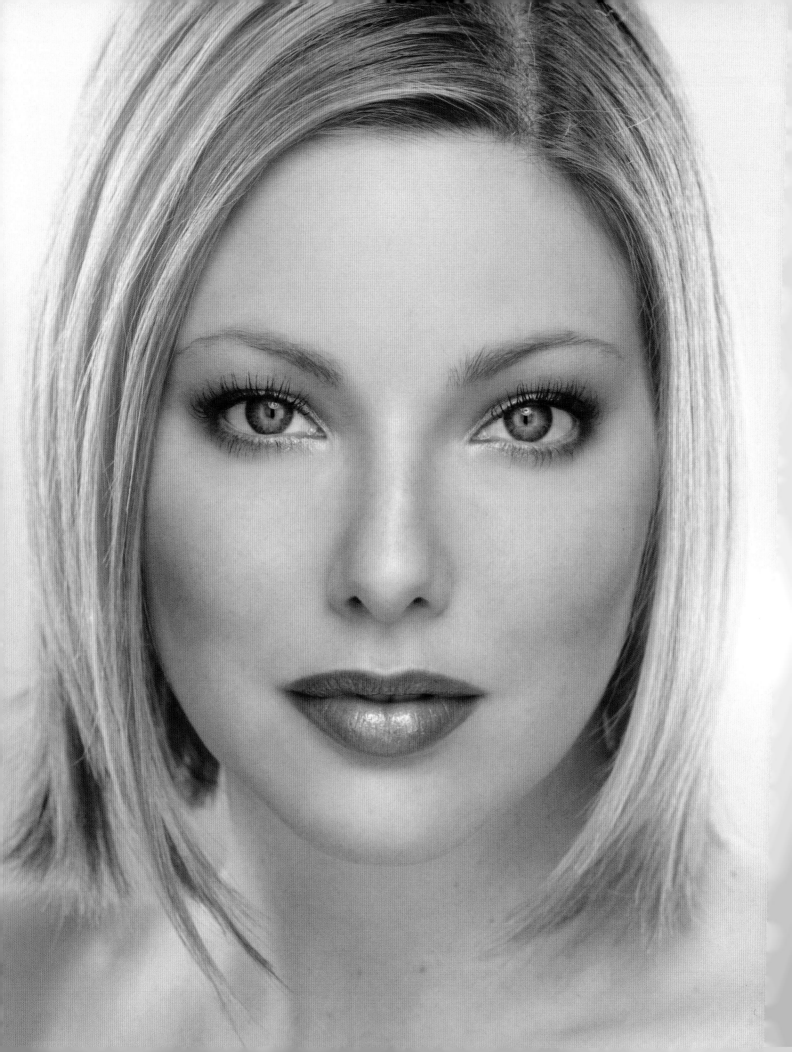

eyes

Three times is definitely a charm when it comes to applying eye color. It takes three shades to shape the eye: a highlight, midtone, and contour shade. The basic rule to remember is that everything you highlight will come toward you or become more prominent, and everything you contour or darken will recede or move away from you. Using three shades creates a subtle visual trick to help bring out one of your most beautiful features and help draw attention to your eyes rather than your eyelids. While there are thousands of shades to choose from, everyone should use the three-shade application technique for best results. Be sure to review pages 111-121 to identify your particular eye shape and learn the correct placement for your three shades.

HIGHLIGHT

Your highlight shade is the lightest of the three eye-shadows. It can be more or less dramatic, depending on the shade and the finish you select. A matte finish will give you a more subtle look than a shimmer finish. The shimmer will be more dramatic. For example, I usually use a shimmer highlight on deep-set eyes because it opens up the eye more than a matte shade. Also, the lighter the highlight shade, the more dramatic your look. A softer or flesh-toned shade will give you a less dramatic look. You should apply the highlight shade to your browbone and eyelid.

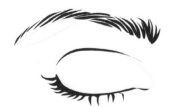 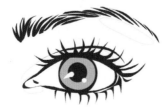

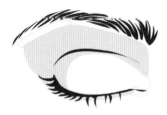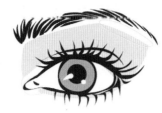

MIDTONE

Your midtone shade is your most important shade. It's the first step in the blending process and in creating the crease of the eye. This shade should be the most subtle—an extension of your skin. You'll change your highlight and contour colors more often than your midtone shade. Most of the time it is best for your midtone color to have a matte finish, but it does not always have to. It is just that the matte finish gives it a more subtle and natural appearance.

To apply it, start from the outside corner of the eyelid, so that area will get the most midtone color. Gently move your brush across the crease into the inside corner of the eyelid. Depending on your eye shape (if yours is any other shape than basic), you may not always want to bring the color all the way over to the inside corner. Refer to pages 111-121 for exact placement. If you want a very defined crease, you can apply a few more layers of your midtone shade, always making sure to blend it where it meets the highlight shade.

If you're short on time, just sweep your midtone color across your eyelids for a very natural look. It will help your eye color "pop," but won't help to define or shape your eyelids.

CONTOUR

The contour shade is the deepest of the three shades. It's not necessarily stark or dark—it can even be metallic—but it is the eyeshadow that is the deepest of the three. The contour eyeshadow is the shade you can have fun with and change with your mood. You'll find that most makeup lines offer more contour colors, because they are the most eye-catching and exciting to use.

To apply, take a brush with shadow and move it across your top lash line from the outside corner inward. Then bring the color up into the outer portion of the crease and blend it inward. This layers the contour shade on top of your midtone shade to help you get the blended, defined look you want. You can also apply the contour color underneath the lower lash line to define or blend it over your eye pencil.

For a more dramatic eye, you can always apply several layers of color to build the shade's intensity. Add color in small amounts. You can always add more for extra drama, but once you've applied it, it's difficult to remove. You can also create a "smoky" eye using your contour color over the entire lid, beginning at the lash line and blending it as you go upwards. For a true smoky look, you must blend, blend, and blend some more, otherwise your eyeshadow will appear too harsh. For more information, see page 221.

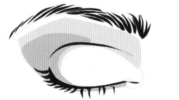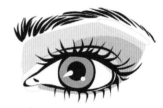

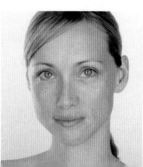

amy williams

EYELINER

You can line and define your eyes in a number of ways: with pencil, liquid, cake, crème, or powder. Or you can skip this step completely! It's a matter of personal choice.

Pencil eyeliners contain silicone to help the color glide on smoothly and blend easily. Make sure the pencil you use doesn't have too much silicone, or the color will smear and smudge underneath your eyes rather than define them.

To apply pencil liner, begin at the outside corner of your eye and draw small, feather-like strokes, connecting each one as you move toward the inside of the eye. Then blend with a small brush. Using the same brush, apply a powder shadow in a similar color over the pencil to help make it look more natural. I always do this because it softens the pencil line and sets the color. It also helps you correct any mistakes you may have made when blending the pencil strokes together.

For nighttime drama, I like to use a pencil underneath the eye and along the upper lash line. Along the upper lashline, make sure the line gradually grows thicker as it extends toward the outer corner of the eyes. Underneath the eye, you want the color to be the most intense at the outer corner and slowly fading as it reaches the inner corner. Drawing the same thickness all the way across and underneath the eyelids can close in the eyes and make them appear smaller. For daytime, I normally don't use pencil underneath the eye. Instead, I like to use an eyeshadow and a brush to create a softer, more natural look. If you prefer to wear pencil during the daytime, be sure to soften it by applying powder over it to make it appear more subtle.

Some women have a more noticeable rim of skin that is visible between the lashes and the eye, depending on their eye shape. You can darken this area with a pencil or a dark shadow to help your eye color "pop." One of my favorite tricks is to take black eyeshadow and carefully push it into the base of the lashes using a fine-tipped brush. This defines the eyes and makes the lashes look thicker without making your eyes appear "lined."

Tips:

You could also use a blush for your midtone if the product has been approved for the eye.

A quick note: The first place you put your brush will receive the most color, because it has the most eyeshadow on it at that point.

Since blending is so vital to the overall effect of beautifully painted eyes, good-quality shadow brushes are a must, because they enable you to create artful shapes and effects.

You should apply concealer and powder to your lids first before applying eyeshadow. This helps the color blend more easily and wear longer.

Always keep your pencils sharpened for more precise application.

Liquid eyeliner is the longest-wearing, and most brands come with a fine-tipped application brush. Liquid liner creates the strongest, most dramatic line. Never use liquid liner under the eye, because it leaves an unnatural line that can be stark and hard-looking.

When using liquid eyeliner on the top of your eyelid, draw a continuous line starting at the inside corner to the outside corner of the eye, giving the line a little "kick" upwards at the end. Make sure it is the most narrow at the inside corner, gradually getting thicker as you get to the outside corner. Liquid eyeliner is the most difficult to apply, but you can master it with a little practice.

Crème eyeliner is also applied with a damp brush in the same manner as liquid and cake.

Cake eyeliner comes as a powder. To apply, first dampen your brush, then swipe it across the powder to form a liquid. Then apply it just as you would liquid eyeliner.

Powder eyeliner, or eyeshadow used as liner, gives the most natural look and is the easiest to work with. You can use it dry, or use it wet if you want a stronger look. To apply it dry, use a brush and draw a fine line along the base of the lashes from the outside to the inside corner of the eye. If you'd like to apply the powder wet, dampen your brush and apply it like liquid eyeliner. Powder used wet gives the same effect as liquid, but is much easier to control.

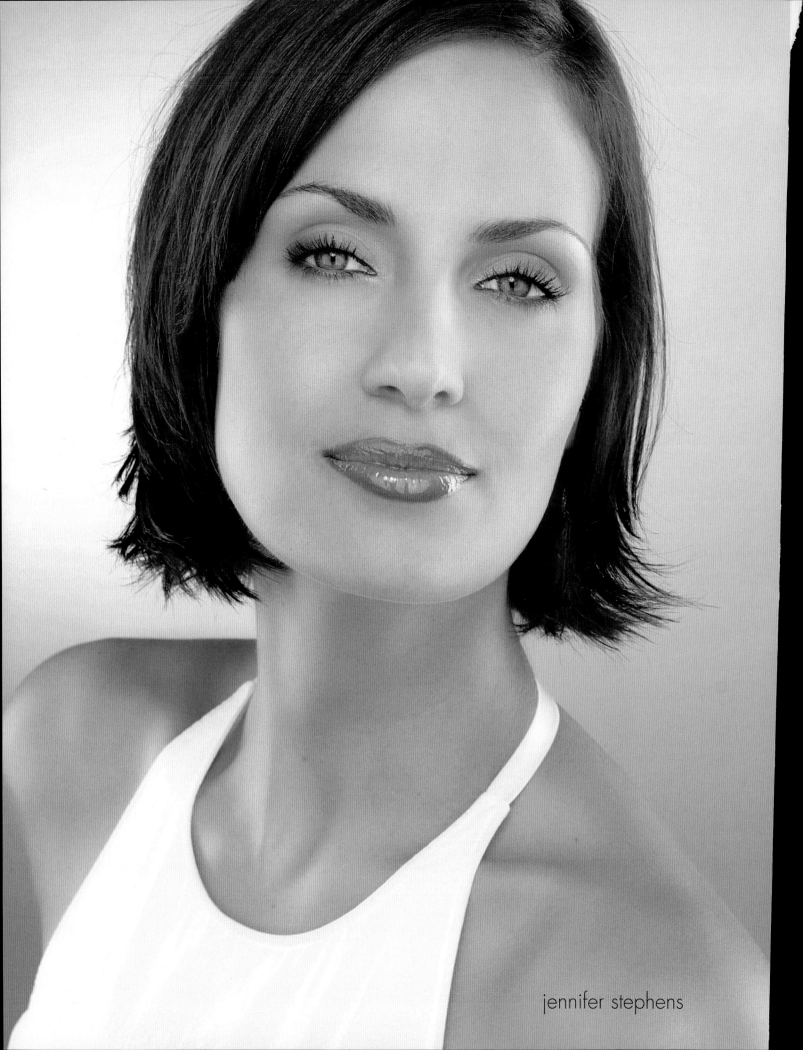

jennifer stephens

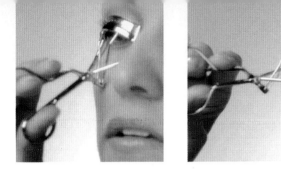 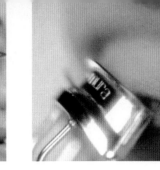 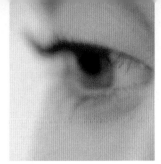

long lashes

I always recommend curling your eyelashes, because it opens up the eyes and makes them appear larger and more youthful. Many women skip this step and it's a mistake. You're never too old to curl your lashes. But make sure the tool you use is young. If you use an eyelash curler for more than a year, it can get out of alignment and cut your lashes.

The trick to curling your eyelashes correctly is to crimp them more than just once at the lash line. Instead, "walk" the eyelash curler up the length of your lashes, taking care to close, open and move the eyelash curler up several times until you reach the end of your lashes. This method creates a curve rather than a crimp, and will help your eyelashes stay curled.

You can make your lashes look longer or thicker by applying your mascara correctly. Thickening and lengthening mascaras contain particles that attach to the lash so you can control how you want to build your lashes.

For thicker lashes: Start at the base of the lashes and hold your mascara wand in a horizontal position, working it from side to side as you work your way up to the end of the lashes. This makes the mascara particles attach to the sides of your lashes, making them appear thicker.

For longer lashes: Hold your mascara wand in a vertical position. Starting at the base of the lash line, pull the wand up and out to the end of your lashes. The particles will attach to the ends of your lashes, making them appear longer.

Make sure you choose the correct formula for your desired effect. If you want to define your lashes, use a defining formula. If you want to thicken, use a thickening formula. Turn to page 32 for more information on the different mascara formulas that are available.

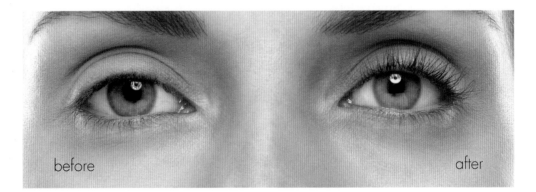

before

after

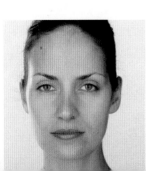

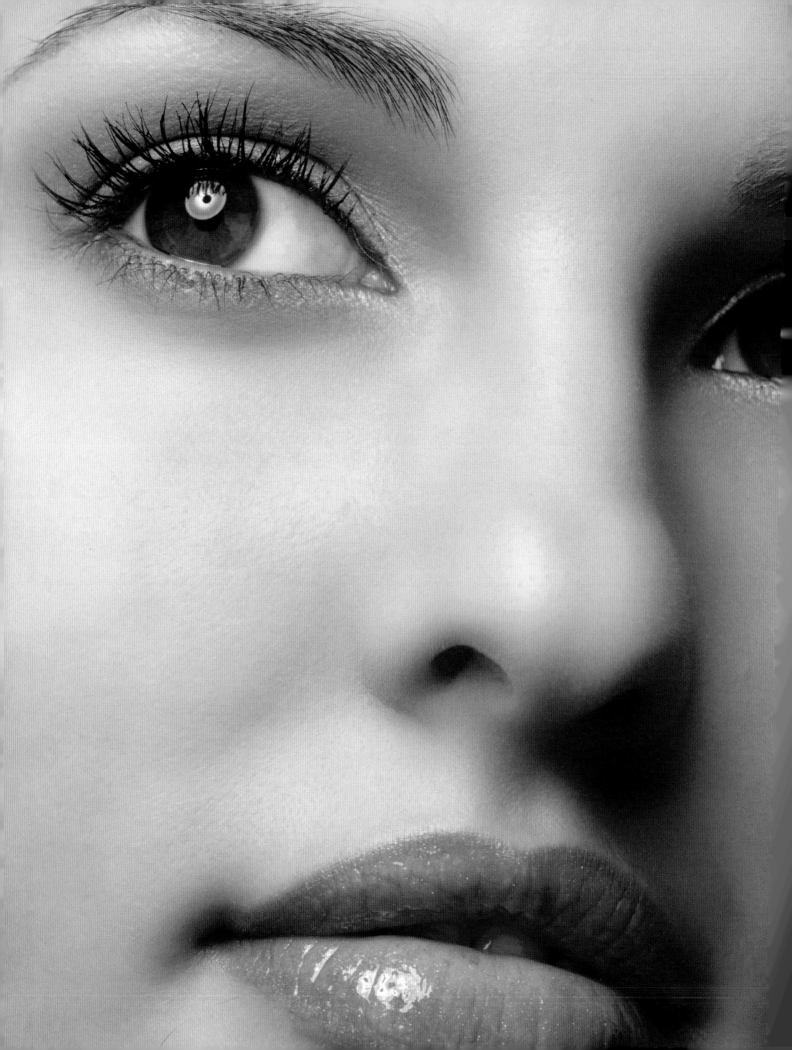

false eyelashes

If you want more drama, you can always wear false eyelashes. They come in **strips, individual flares, and individual strands.**

If you'd like that flirtatious, "frankly fake" look for evening, use the strips, because they are the most noticeable.

It's best to apply a pencil eyeliner before your strip eyelashes so you can see exactly where to place them, and to prevent any skin from showing between your natural lashes and the false ones. The closer you place them to your natural lashline, the more natural they'll appear. You can follow with a liquid liner to help disguise the lash band.

The flares are more natural-looking than strips, but my preference is for the individual-strand lashes. They look the most natural, and they are the ones typically used for most mascara advertisements. You simply apply them directly on top of your own lashes to help extend the length.

Tips:

I personally prefer to use black mascara on the upper lashes and brown on the lower ones, because brown looks less harsh.

Make certain you coat your lashes with mascara at the inside corners and the very outer corners. These are the two areas that many women miss.

Two or three thinly applied coats of mascara are far more effective than a single clumpy one.

cheek chic

Blush and bronzer work together to bring your face alive and give you a natural, healthy glow. Getting that beautiful glow is a two-step process, because I always like to bronze the face before adding the actual cheek color. I think every woman can benefit from bronzing because it adds warmth and natural beauty to the skin and can make you appear younger.

Before we learn how to bronze and blush correctly, I want to shatter the old myths of where and how to apply color to your cheeks.

Myth 1: *Blush should never be worn closer to your nose than the width of two fingers.* Depending on the width of your fingers, your blush could wind up on the side of your face instead of the apples of your cheeks!

Myth 2: *Blush should never be applied below the tip of your nose.* If you followed this advice and you have a cute little turned-up nose, your blush could be applied above the apples of your cheeks.

Myth 3: *Apply blush as an inverted triangle to the face to give it more shape.* We use foundation and powder to highlight and contour the face—not blush. Blush is used to add color and life to the skin.

Myth 4: *Mature women should apply cheek color higher as they age.* While the skin may lose some of its elasticity as we age, I can assure you that our cheekbones remain in the same place! If you know how to locate your cheekbones correctly, you'll always have your bronzer and blush in the right place on your face.

To accurately locate your cheekbones, take this can't-miss application test:

1. Smile.

2. Locate the center of the "apple" of your cheek and place your index finger there. Next, place your thumb at the top of your ear where it connects to your head. Now take your thumb and bring it toward your index finger. The bone you feel is your cheekbone. Finally, apply your color directly onto the cheekbone.

Tip:

Keep separate brushes for bronzers and blush, because it keeps each color clearer and purer.

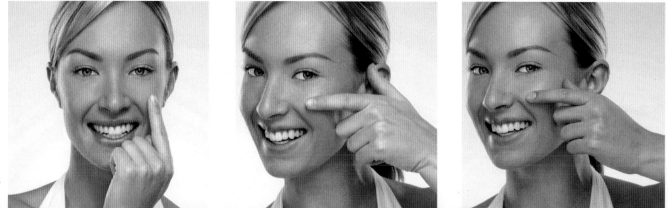

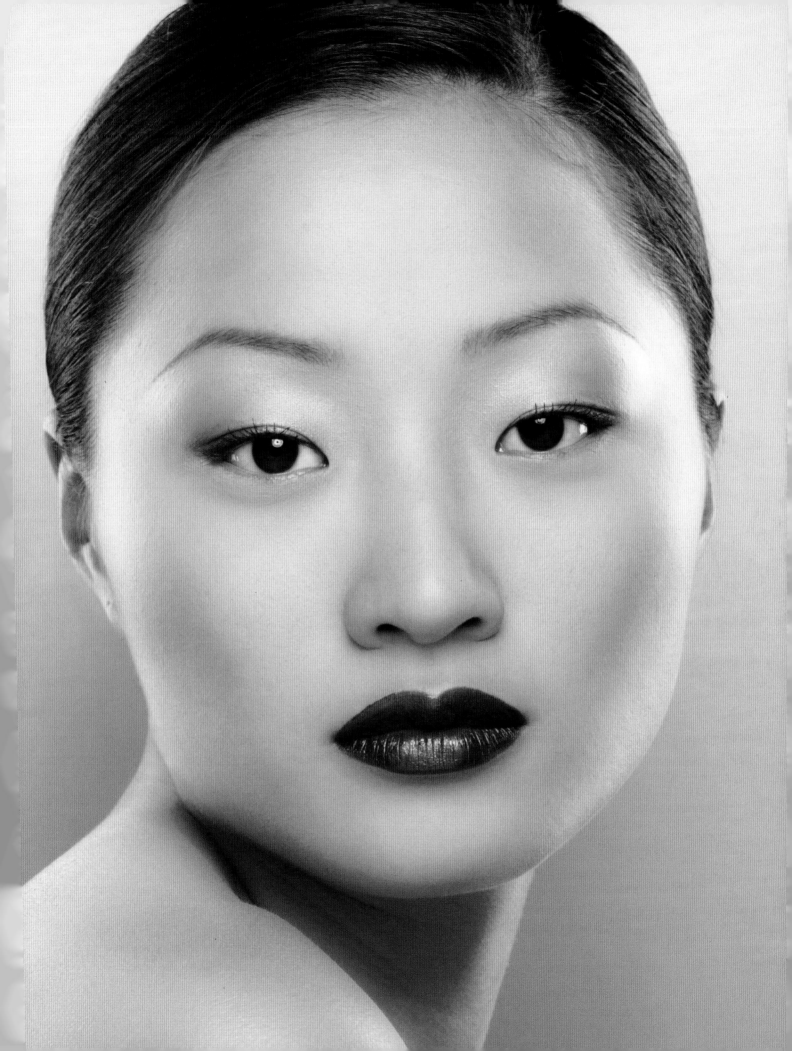

BRONZER

Bronzer makes your skin look sun-kissed and alive. It gives your skin a healthy glow without subjecting it to damaging ultraviolet rays. To warm your face and accentuate your bone structure, simply dust bronzing powder or crème bronzer along the outer edges of your face and onto your cheekbones. Bronzer is also useful for lightly sculpting the nose and chin. See page 83 for more info on sculpting.

Always apply your bronzer beginning at the back of your cheekbone and sweep it forward. Then go back and brush in the opposite direction to blend. If you are using a crème bronzer, simply dot the color along your cheekbone and blend. Don't forget a little at the temples to help shape your face. Sweeping the bronzing powder up around the temples and eye sockets can also really help your eye color pop, especially if your eyes are green or blue.

If bronzing powders and crèmes look too bold on you, try using pressed powder instead. It has a lower pigment level and blends very nicely. If you have lighter skin, an ebony pressed powder will work beautifully as a bronzer.

BLUSH

There are three major mistakes women make with blush:

1. Using too much of it in the fall and winter to try to compensate for the lack of a tan.

2. Choosing a color that is either too red or too purple. Remember, to help determine a good shade for yourself, try a short burst of energetic exercise, then match your blush color to your cheeks' natural flush.

3. Applying too little of a shade because it's too strong. If you don't apply enough, it won't last through the day.

The intensity of color you are wearing on your eyes and lips can determine the amount of blush you might need that day. For example, if you are wearing a strong lip color, you will need less blush. If you are wearing a paler, sheerer lip color, you might need more blush.

A powder blush is the easiest to use. There are two ways to apply your powder blush properly:

1. Apply blush to your cheekbone area, starting at the back (closest to your ear). Sweep your cheek color toward the apple of your cheek, then back toward the ear again. Then go back again in the opposite direction to blend. This way, your most intense color lies at the back of your cheek and gives your face more dimension.

2. For a more natural appearance, you can try a technique called "popping your apples." First, apply bronzer to your cheekbones. Then take a light, sheer blush color, making sure it is not too dark. Smile and apply your blush color back toward the area that you bronzed. This gives the apples of your cheeks a beautiful glow. Again, you'll want to use a sheer shade of blush for this technique. A dark or bright cheek color can be too intense and unnatural-looking.

If you use crème or liquid blush, apply it with either a sponge or your fingers after your foundation and before your powder for easier blending. If you wear your blush without foundation, crème and liquid work better than powder blush as they contain moisture that blends better with the natural moisture of your skin. To apply crème or liquid blush, first dot a little onto the apples of your cheeks and then blend back toward your ears.

With any blush, you should remember the rule to match textures: crème on crème and powder on powder. To increase the staying power of your blush, try these tips:

1. Apply crème blush after you apply your foundation.

2. Apply your pressed or loose powder.

3. Apply powder blush on top of your face powder. The two layers help the cheek color stay on and last throughout the day.

Tips:

If cheek color is too intense, soften it with a dusting of loose powder.

Never use blush to contour or shape the face.

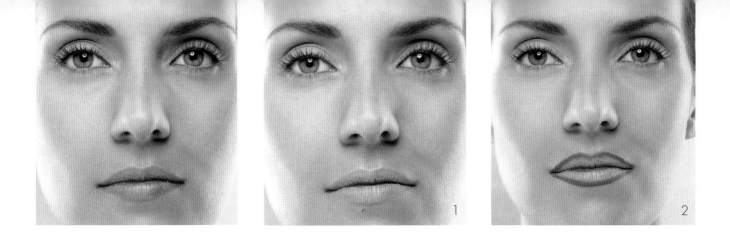

lips

To keep your lips looking luscious, exfoliate them once a week. I always like to use a little lip balm or moisturizer on the lips before I apply the lipstick color, because it helps the lip liner and lipstick go on smoothly and more evenly. Just apply the lip balm first and blot off the excess.

Lip pencils will help prevent lipstick from feathering and bleeding, but once you've outlined your lips, don't stop there. Be sure to blend inward so that when your lipstick wears off, you aren't left with just an outline. You'll find a brush useful in the application and blending.

Make sure you optimize your entire mouth. Most women don't, because they tend to draw inside the lip line. Conversely, take care not to overdraw, because if you're using a lip color that is not natural-looking and you stray too far outside the lip line, it will be noticeable.

BASIC

I'm often asked if women have to wear lip liner. While it's an optional step, here are three things to consider to help you decide if lip liner is for you:

1. Lip liner can help define your mouth and reshape your lips if they are uneven.

2. Lip liner can help prevent your lip color from bleeding onto your skin.

3. Lip liner can help your lipstick last longer, especially if you fill in your lips with liner first before applying your lip color.

APPLICATION:

To properly apply your lip liner to the top lip, begin with a V in the "cupid's bow" or center curve of the lips. Then starting at the outer corners, draw small, feathery strokes to meet the center V.

On the lower lip, first accentuate the lower curve of the lip, then begin small feather-like strokes from the outer corners moving towards the center.

Now you can actually apply your color. You can use a brush, your fingers, or a tube to apply your lipstick, but if it's applied with a brush, it will usually look much more precise and last longer. For more intense color, you can apply it straight from the tube, but it will be harder to cover the smaller detailed areas of the lips.

SMALL LIPS

If you feel you have small lips, there are two ways to create a new, fuller lip look. Here's the first way:

1. First, erase your existing lip line with concealer or foundation. Doing this creates a fresh canvas on which you can design a whole new and improved lip line.

2. Using a natural-toned lip pencil, draw a line just slightly above your natural lip line on the top and around the bottom. Don't exaggerate the line—just slightly above and below your natural lip line is your goal.

3. Now, fill in your lips completely with the lip liner, except for the very center of your top lip and bottom lip.

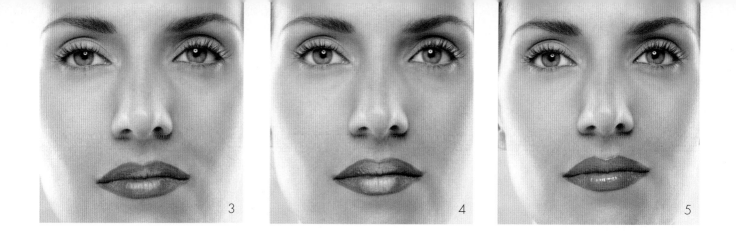

3

4

5

4. Next, take a dab of light concealer and place it in the center of your top lip and bottom lip. When you apply your lipstick, this area will remain lighter and help make your lips appear fuller.

5. To finish, apply a light, shimmery lip gloss to the center of your lips over your lipstick to help make your lips appear even fuller.

The second way to create fuller lips is by using two complementary shades of lip color—one lighter, one darker. First, line your lips with a natural-toned lip pencil. Then apply the darker shade of lip color on the outer edges of your lips, blending it where it meets the lip liner. Next, apply the lighter shade of lipstick on the inside of your lips and blend it where it meets the darker shade. Finally, take a light, shimmery lip gloss and place it in the center of the lips to create the illusion of fuller lips.

Choosing the correct formula for the desired lip look is important. Glossy is always sexy. The shine makes your lips appear fuller and more youthful. If your lips tend to be dry, stay away from matte lipstick. While the formula wears longer, it can make your lips look and feel even more dehydrated. Crème formulas are always a safe choice, because they tend to work in just about any situation.

Play with lip color. Don't be afraid of it. It's always easy to change it. Just remember it's important to consider your lip size when choosing a lipstick color. Darker shades make the lips look smaller. Lighter shades make the lips look fuller. To review the guidelines for choosing lip color, turn to page 67.

One last point to remember: Never expect lipstick to last all day. Formulas that last that long make the lips look parched and dry. These products contain stains that (unless your lips are freshly exfoliated) will adhere unevenly to the dry areas of your lips, causing your lipstick to appear splotchy and dehydrated.

Tips:

Don't forget that brighter, warmer colors also make you look younger. Anything too dark is far too harsh for mature lips.

Remember that paler colors illuminate and make lips appear fuller and more youthful, while dark colors have a minimizing effect, making lips appear smaller.

Always moisturize your lips before applying color.

To help lipstick stay on longer, use lip liner all over your lips. Apply lipstick on top, then blot and reapply.

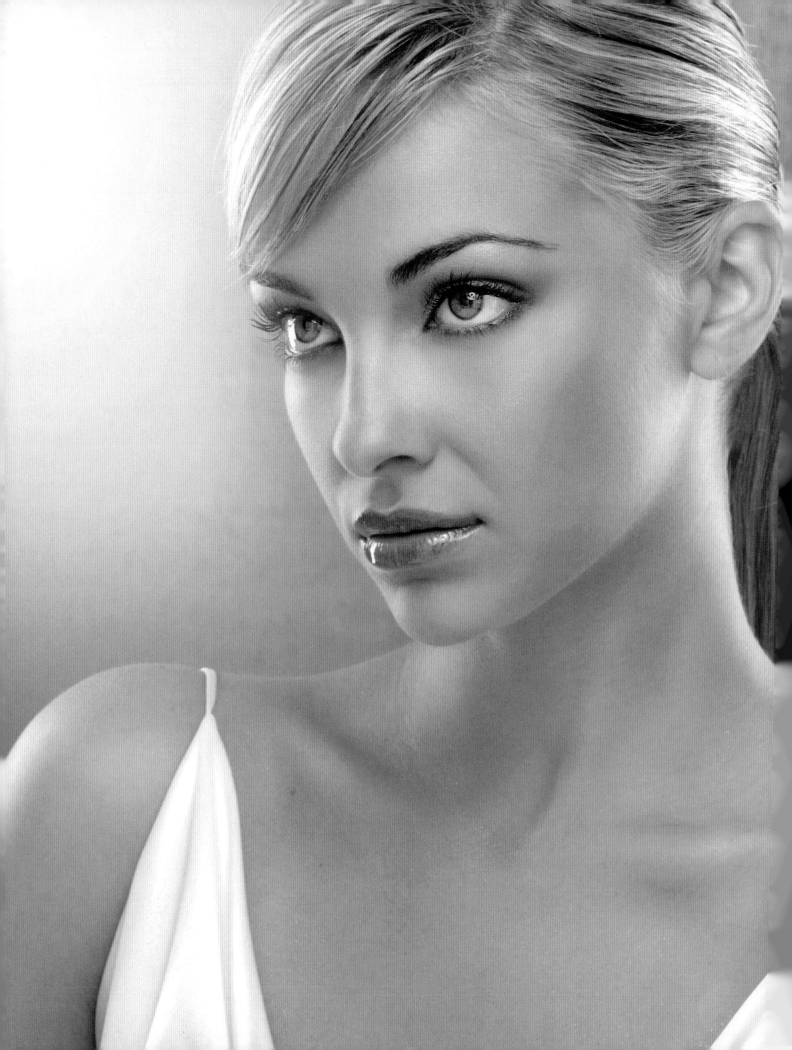

totaltransformations

I have already stated that every woman is beautiful, and in this chapter I prove it! I have taken women from every walk of life, ethnic background, and age, and shown how beautiful they all truly are. Enjoy seeing the transformations and the tips about how I achieved each look. I am sure that with such a diverse group of women, even you can find someone with a similar look and will be able to take the application tips and use them to make yourself more beautiful. Just remember, makeup is not permanent, so don't be scared to try new things. If you do not like it when you are finished, you can just wash it off. Have fun and become your most beautiful you!

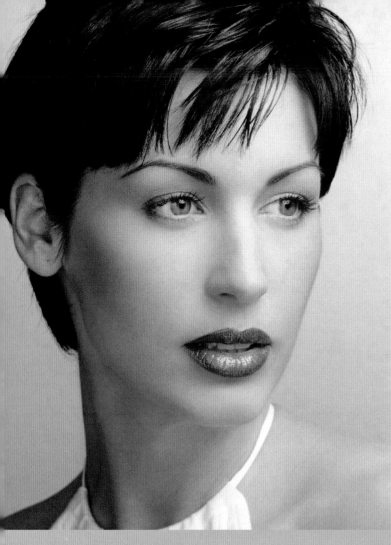

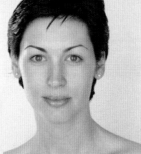

kerrie bodrato

FACE SHAPE: oval
EYE SHAPE: basic
SHADOWS: Highlight: shimmer flesh
        Midtone: matte taupe
        Contour: shimmer golden brown
OBJECTIVE: To add contrast and color to her face. To open the eyes and create a more defined crease.
APPLICATION: Chose lip and blush colors that were in great contrast to her skin to add color to her face. Defined her eyes really well at the lash line. Made sure to define the crease really well with my midtone so as to deepen it and add shape to her eye and lid.

lana andrews

FACE SHAPE: square
EYE SHAPE: deep-set
SHADOWS: Highlight: shimmer gold
        Midtone: matte taupe
        Contour: shimmer golden brown
OBJECTIVE: To create the illusion of a more oval-shaped face. To bring her eyes out and push browbone back.
APPLICATION: Contoured the hairline and jaw to soften the "four corners" of the face. Highlighted the center of the forehead, nose, and tip of the chin. Highlighted lid only, to bring the eye forward. Used midtone on browbone to push it away.

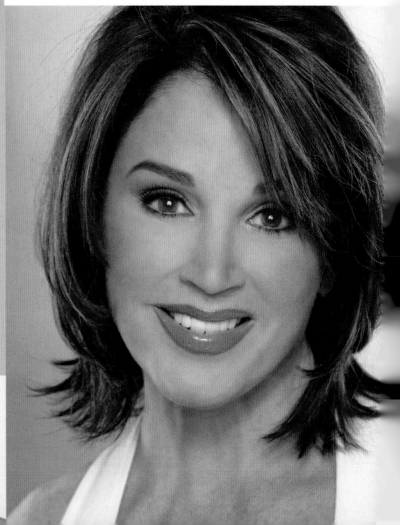

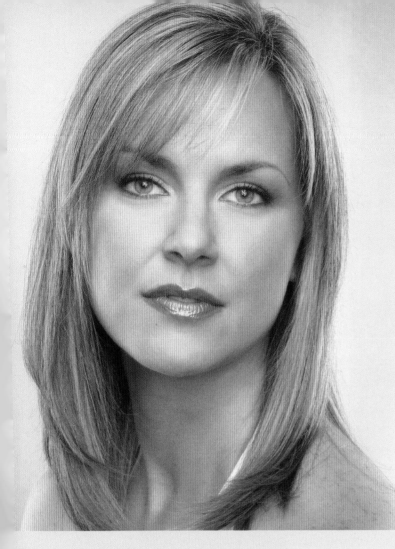

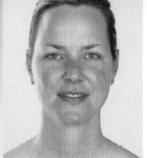

gayle kolsrud

FACE SHAPE: square
EYE SHAPE: basic
SHADOWS: Highlight: shimmer flesh
Midtone: matte taupe
Contour: shimmer golden brown
OBJECTIVE: To create the illusion of a more oval-shaped face and to subtly define her features.
APPLICATION: Contoured the hairline and jaw to soften the "four corners" of the face. Highlighted the center of the forehead, nose, and tip of the chin. Highlighted the lid and browbone to open up the eye. Defined the crease and lash line to give the eye more shape.

pat smith

FACE SHAPE: square
EYE SHAPE: basic
SHADOWS: Highlight: shimmer gold
Midtone: matte mahogany
Contour: matte dark brown
OBJECTIVE: To give the illusion of a more oval-shaped face.
APPLICATION: Contoured the hairline and jaw to soften the "four corners" of the face. Highlighted down the center of the forehead, nose, and tip of the chin. Highlighted the lid and browbone. To create definition at the lash line and in the crease, chose to layer the midtone color rather than a darker color.

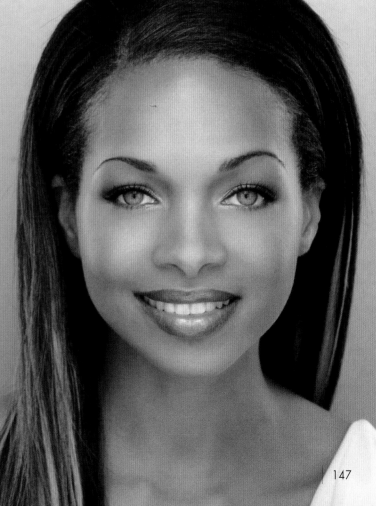

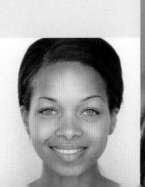

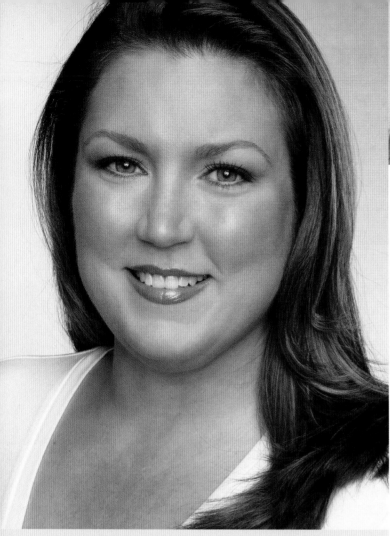

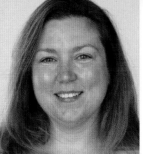

tracey allred

FACE SHAPE: pear
EYE SHAPE: basic
SHADOWS: Highlight: shimmer flesh
              Midtone: matte rose
              Contour: shimmer golden brown
OBJECTIVE: To create the illusion of a more oval-shaped face. Highlight and open her eyes which are one of her best features.
APPLICATION: Contoured jawline and cheeks to help minimize their width. Highlighted the center of the forehead to create the illusion of more width. Highlighted eyelids and browbones to open the eyes. Defined the crease and lash line.

gloria mayfield-banks

FACE SHAPE: oval
EYE SHAPE: droopy
SHADOWS: Highlight: shimmer gold
              Midtone: matte mahogany
              Contour: matte burgundy
OBJECTIVE: To even out skin tone and brighten areas to add life to the skin. To make the outer corners of the eyes appear to turn up rather than down.
APPLICATION: To even out the skin tone, used multiple shades of foundation then brightened the skin with a golden orange face powder on all highlight areas of the face. Made sure to begin all midtone and contour shadow application in slightly from the outside corner of the eye, making sure to blend up and in, not out and down.

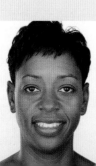

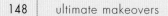

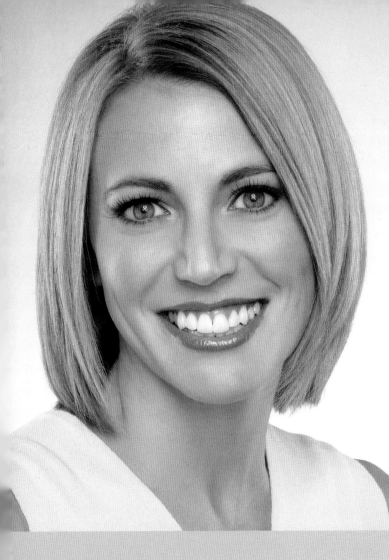

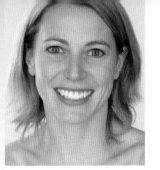

susan porter glassmoyer

FACE SHAPE: oval
EYE SHAPE: hooded
SHADOWS: Highlight: shimmer beige
          Midtone: matte taupe
          Contour: shimmer golden brown
OBJECTIVE: To contour the lid to draw attention
to her eyes.
APPLICATION: Layered midtone and contour colors on
hooded areas. The layering of color helps the end result
appear more subtle and natural.

brooke tobolka

FACE SHAPE: square
EYE SHAPE: basic
SHADOWS: Highlight: shimmer beige
          Midtone: matte taupe
          Contour: matte dark brown
OBJECTIVE: To create the illusion of a more
oval-shaped face.
APPLICATION: Contoured the hairline and jaw to soften
the "four corners" of the face. Highlighted down the center
of the forehead, nose, and tip of the chin. Brooke has
slightly hooded lids, so I applied and blended midtone
and contour colors to the area to help it recede. Defined
the lash line really well.

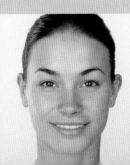

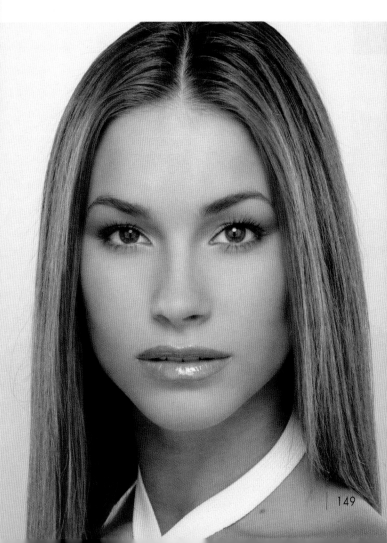

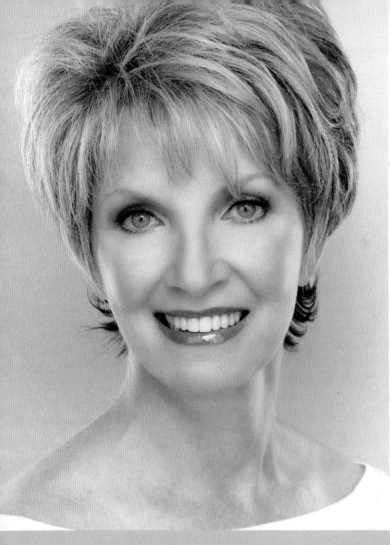

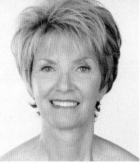

arlene lenarz

FACE SHAPE: square
EYE SHAPE: wide-set
SHADOWS: Highlight: shimmer flesh
                Midtone: matte taupe
                Contour: shimmer golden brown
OBJECTIVE: To give the illusion of a more oval-shaped
face and help the eyes appear closer together.
APPLICATION: Contoured the hairline and jaw to soften
the "four corners" of the face. Highlighted down the center
of the forehead, nose, and tip of the chin. Layered midtone
color in the crease and on the inside hollow of the eye to
visually pull the eye placement closer together.

roshawnda r. foster

FACE SHAPE: pear
EYE SHAPE: basic
SHADOWS: Highlight: shimmer gold
                Midtone: matte mahogany
                Contour: dark burgundy
OBJECTIVE: To create the illusion of a more
oval-shaped face.
APPLICATION: Contoured the temples and defined the
hollows of the cheeks to help minimize the width of those
areas. Highlighted the chin to create the illusion of width.
Highlighted the lid and browbone to open the eye. Used
midtone shadow to even out her lids, then defined the lash
line really well.

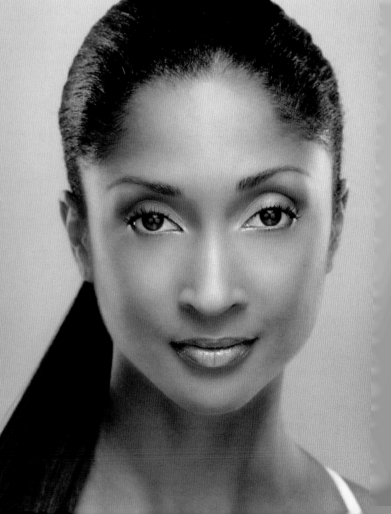

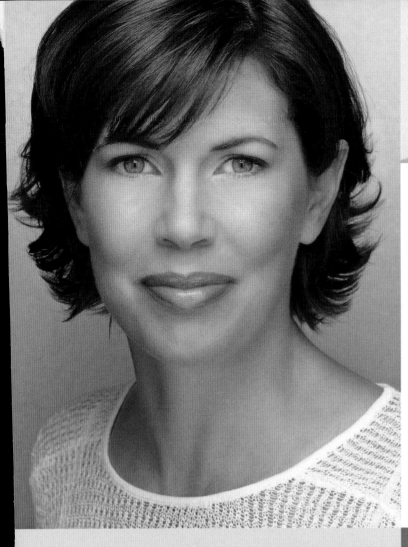

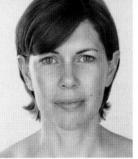

susan t. billy

FACE SHAPE: oval
EYE SHAPE: hooded
SHADOWS: Highlight: shimmer beige
Midtone: matte taupe
Contour: shimmer golden brown
OBJECTIVE: To contour the eyelid away to draw attention to the eyes.
APPLICATION: Layered midtone and contour colors on hooded areas. The layering of color helps the end result appear more subtle and natural.

wanda dalby

FACE SHAPE: oval
EYE SHAPE: hooded
SHADOWS: Highlight: shimmer flesh
Midtone: matte taupe
Contour: shimmer golden brown
OBJECTIVE: To minimize the hooded area and "open up" the eye. To give her skin a youthful glow.
APPLICATION: Applied midtone and contour color to the hooded area of the eyelids to help them recede and "open up" the eye. Subtle layering of color creates a very natural effect. Chose a soft warm blush to give her face a warm glow.

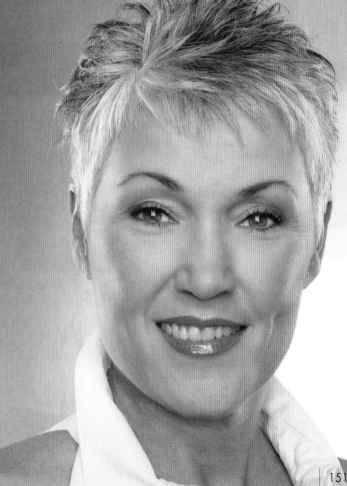

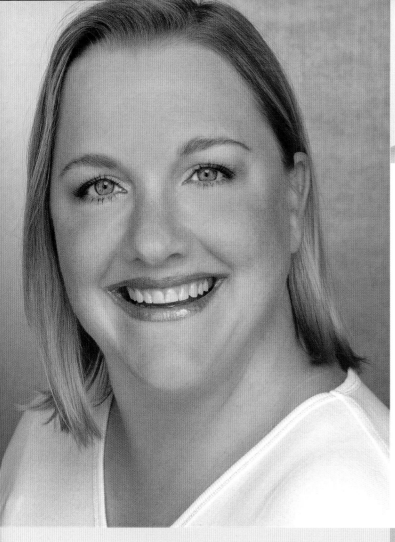

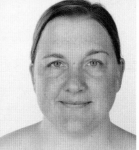

mary diamond

FACE SHAPE: round
EYE SHAPE: hooded
SHADOWS: Highlight: shimmer flesh
               Midtone: matte dark taupe
               Contour-shimmer golden brown
OBJECTIVE: To give the illusion of a more oval-shaped face. To minimize the hooded area and "open up" the eye.
APPLICATION: Softly sculpted cheeks, jaw, and temples to create a more oval shape. Applied midtone and contour color to the hooded area of the lids to help them recede and "open up" the eye. Subtle layering of color creates a very natural effect. A really well-defined lash line makes the blue in her eyes stand out.

julie baker

FACE SHAPE: square
EYE SHAPE: hooded
SHADOWS: Highlight: shimmer beige
               Midtone: matte taupe
               Contour: matte mahogany
OBJECTIVE: To give the illusion of a more oval-shaped face. To minimize the hooded appearance of her eyelids, making her eyes appear more open and alive.
APPLICATION: Contoured the hairline and jaw to soften the "four corners" of the face. Highlighted down the center of the forehead, nose, and tip of the chin. I applied, then blended the midtone and contour colors onto the hooded area to help it appear to recede.

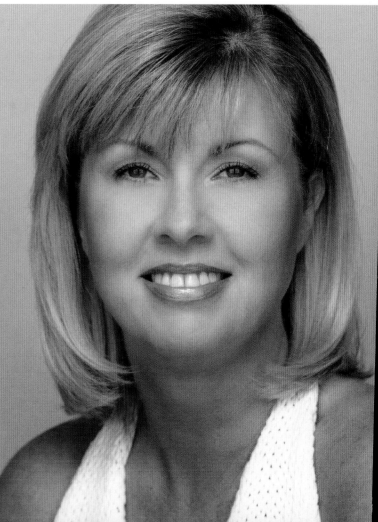

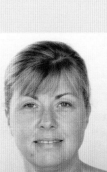

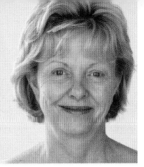

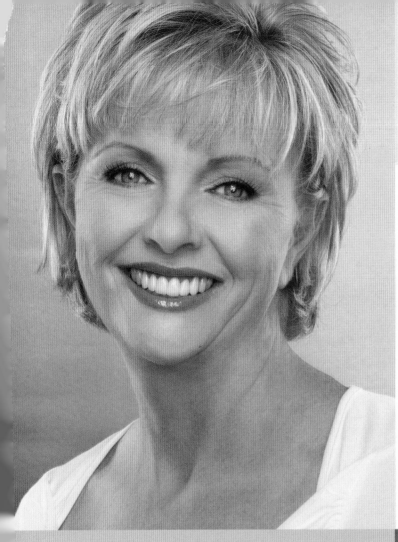

lynda keene

FACE SHAPE: oval
EYE SHAPE: wide-set
SHADOWS: Highlight: shimmer beige
   Midtone: matte rose
   Contour: matte dark brown
OBJECTIVE: To visually bring the eyes closer together and to give her a youthful glow.
APPLICATION: Layered the color in the crease and on the inside hollows of the eyes to visually pull the eye shape closer together. Used warm lip and cheek shades to give her skin a more youthful glow.

maxine allen

FACE SHAPE: oval
EYE SHAPE: droopy
SHADOWS: Highlight: matte sand
   Midtone: matte caramel
   Contour: matte dark brown
OBJECTIVE: To even out skin tone and brighten areas to help add life to the skin. To make the outer corners of the eye appear to turn up rather than down.
APPLICATION: Evened out skin tone by using multiple shades of foundation. Brightened the skin with a golden-orange face powder on all highlighted areas of the face. Applied the midtone and contour shadows slightly in from the outside corners of the eyes to draw attention to the center of the eyelids. Blended shadows well.

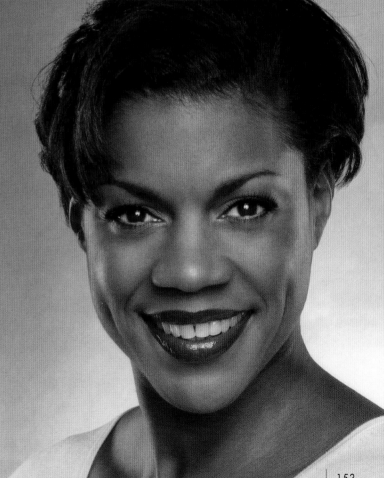

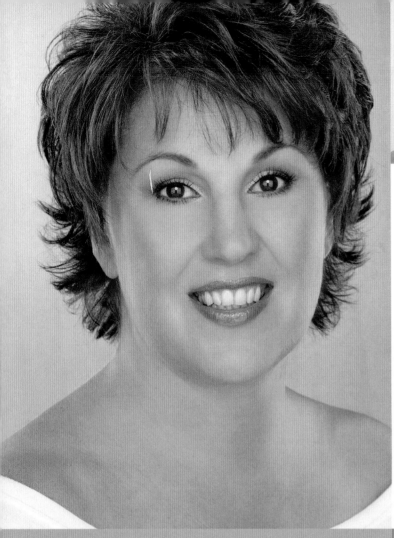

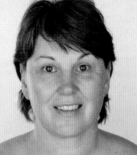

jan harris

FACE SHAPE: pear
EYE SHAPE: basic
SHADOWS: Highlight: shimmer flesh
Midtone: matte taupe
Contour: shimmer golden brown
OBJECTIVE: To give the illusion of a more oval-shaped face. To really define and open up her eyes and make them appear larger.
APPLICATION: Contoured the temples and defined the hollows of the cheeks to help minimize the width of those areas. Highlighted the chin to create the illusion of width. Defined really well with shadow at lash line and by curling her lashes and using multiple layers of mascara. Highlighted lid and inside along bottom lash line to help open her eyes.

nancy castro

FACE SHAPE: square
EYE SHAPE: basic
SHADOWS: Highlight: shimmer beige
Midtone: matte taupe
Contour: matte dark brown
OBJECTIVE: To create the illusion of a more oval-shaped face and to make her eye color "pop."
APPLICATION: Contoured the hairline and jaw to soften the "four corners" of the face. Highlighted the center of the forehead, nose, and tip of the chin. Highlighted the lid and browbone to open up the eye. Defined the crease and lash line to give the eye more shape and to make eye color "pop."

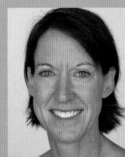

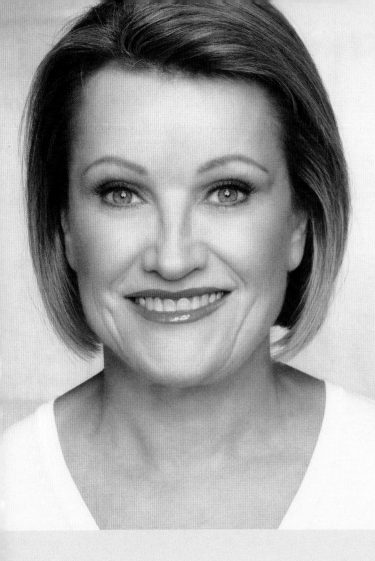

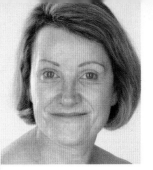

dr. fran kaiser

FACE SHAPE: square
EYE SHAPE: basic
SHADOWS: Highlight: shimmer flesh
Midtone: matte taupe
Contour: shimmer golden brown
OBJECTIVE: To create the illusion of a more oval-shaped face and to give her skin a more youthful glow.
APPLICATION: Contoured the hairline and jaw to soften the "four corners" of the face. Highlighted the center of the forehead, nose, and tip of the chin. Highlighted the lid and browbone to open up the eye. Defined the crease and lashline to give the eye more shape. Chose a soft, warm blush to give her face a warm glow.

sonia paez

FACE SHAPE: pear
EYE SHAPE: hooded
SHADOWS: Highlight: shimmer gold
Midtone: matte dark taupe
Contour: shimmer golden brown
OBJECTIVE: To give the illusion of a more oval-shaped face. To minimize the hooded appearance of her eyelids, making her eyes appear more open.
APPLICATION: Contoured the temples and defined the hollows of the cheeks to help minimize the width of those areas. Highlighted the chin to create the illusion of width. I applied, then blended, the midtone and contour colors onto the hooded area of the eyelids, making them appear to recede.

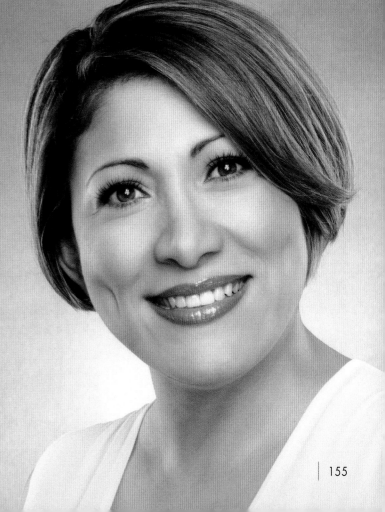

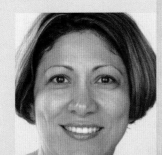

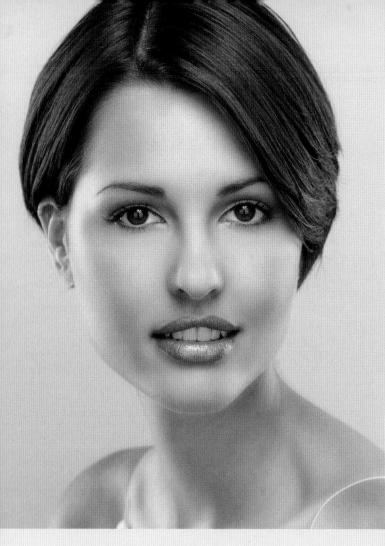

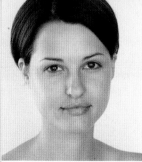

erica tracy

FACE SHAPE: square
EYE SHAPE: basic
SHADOWS: Highlight: shimmer beige
Midtone: matte taupe
Contour: shimmer golden brown
OBJECTIVE: To give the illusion of a more oval-shaped face.
APPLICATION: Contoured hairline and jaw to soften the "four corners" of the face. Highlighted down the center of the forehead, nose, and tip of the chin. Made sure to highlight the lid and browbone to open the eye. Defined the crease and lash line to give the eye more shape.

joanna hathcock

FACE SHAPE: square
EYE SHAPE: basic
SHADOWS: Highlight: shimmer beige
Midtone: matte taupe
Contour: shimmer golden brown
OBJECTIVE: To create the illusion of a more oval-shaped face.
APPLICATION: Contoured the hairline and jaw to soften the "four corners" of the face. Highlighted down the center of the forehead, nose, and tip of the chin to create an oval illusion. Joanna has very unusually shaped eyes. To accentuate them, I highlighted the lid and brow, then built contour color in the crease and at the lash line.

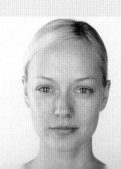

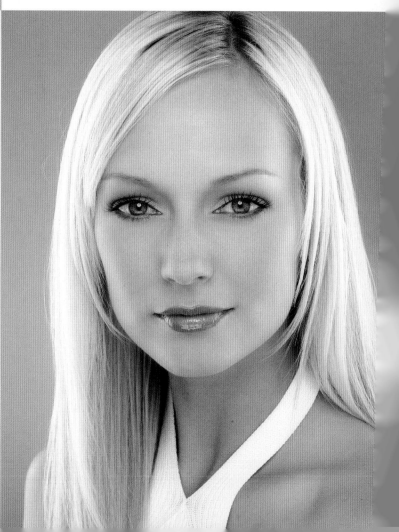

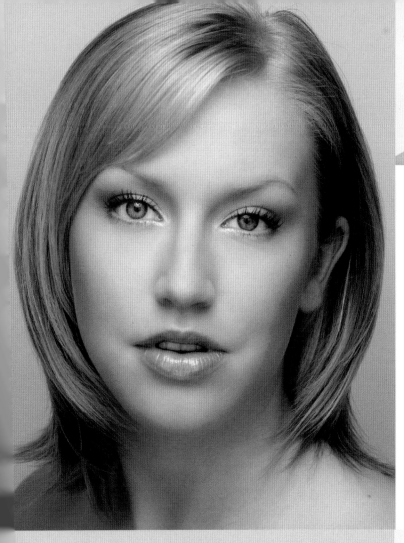

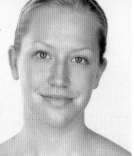

allison piro

FACE SHAPE: heart
EYE SHAPE: basic
SHADOWS: Highlight: shimmer flesh
              Midtone: matte taupe
              Contour: shimmer golden brown
OBJECTIVE: To give the illusion of a more oval-shaped face.
APPLICATION: Contoured her temples and the hollows of her cheeks to minimize the width. Highlighted the chin to create the illusion of more width. Made sure to define the lash line really well to intensify the color of the eyes.

kim henry

FACE SHAPE: square
EYE SHAPE: basic
SHADOWS: Highlight: matte sand
              Midtone: matte mahogany
              Contour: dark burgundy
OBJECTIVE: To even out skin tone and brighten areas to help add life to the skin. To give face a more oval illusion.
APPLICATION: Evened out skin tone by using multiple shades of foundation. Brightened the skin with a golden-orange face powder on all highlighted areas of the face. Contoured the hairline and jaw to soften the "four corners" of the face. Highlighted the center of the forehead, nose, and tip of the chin. Highlighted the lid and browbone to open up the eye. Defined the crease and lash line to give the eye more shape.

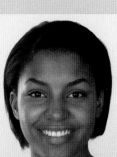

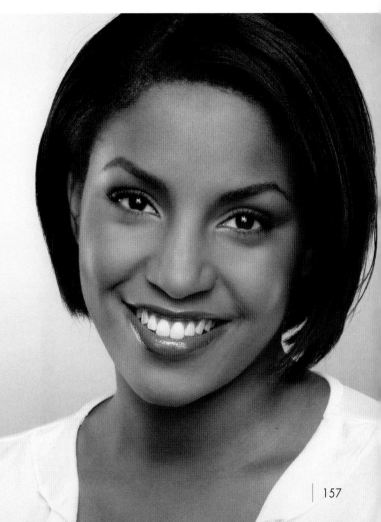

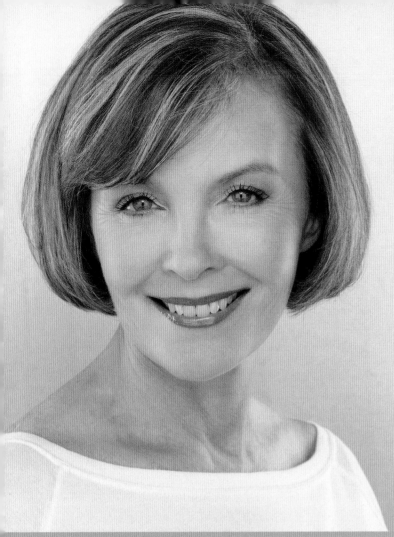

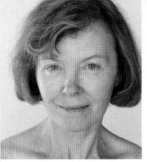

patricia young

FACE SHAPE: oval
EYE SHAPE: droopy
SHADOWS: Highlight: shimmer beige
               Midtone: matte taupe
               Contour: shimmer golden brown
OBJECTIVE: To make the outer corners of the
eyes appear to turn up rather than down. Give
her skin a youthful glow.
APPLICATION: Made sure to begin all midtone
and contour shadow application in slightly from
the outside corner of the eye, making sure to blend up
and in, not out and down. Chose a soft, warm blush
to give her face a warm glow.

sarah bird

FACE SHAPE: pear
EYE SHAPE: basic
SHADOWS: Highlight: shimmer beige
               Midtone: matte taupe
               Contour: matte dark taupe
OBJECTIVE: To give the illusion of a more oval-shaped
face and subtly define her features without making her
look too mature.
APPLICATION: Contoured the jawline and cheeks to help
minimize their width. Highlighted the forehead to create
the illusion of more width. Subtly defined her eyes at the
lash line and highlighted her lids and browbones.

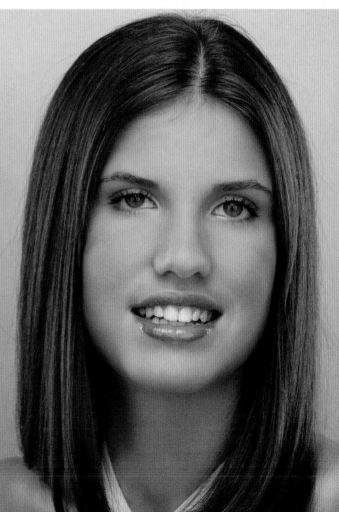

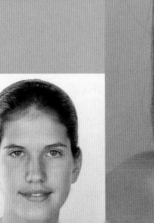

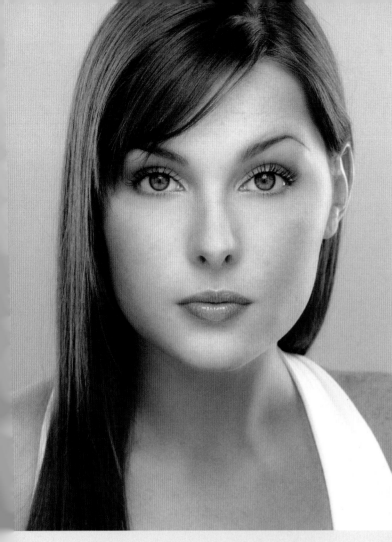

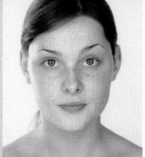

ashley cantley

FACE SHAPE: pear
EYE SHAPE: basic
SHADOWS: Highlight: shimmer beige
              Midtone: matte taupe
              Contour: shimmer golden brown
OBJECTIVE: To give the illusion of a more oval-shaped face and draw more attention to the eyes.
APPLICATION: Contoured the jawline and the hollows of the cheeks to help minimize their width. Highlighted the center of the forehead to help create width. To help bring attention to the eyes, defined the lash line and the crease really well.

holly jonsson

FACE SHAPE: square
EYE SHAPE: basic
SHADOWS: Highlight: shimmer flesh
              Midtone: matte taupe
              Contour: matte dark taupe
OBJECTIVE: To give the illusion of a more oval-shaped face. To define her features without the use of a lot of color.
APPLICATION: Contoured the hairline and jaw to soften the "four corners" of the face. Highlighted down the center of the forehead, nose, and the tip of the chin. I wanted a minimal look so I used much more subtle colors to define, therefore giving her a practically no-makeup look.

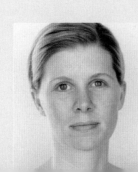

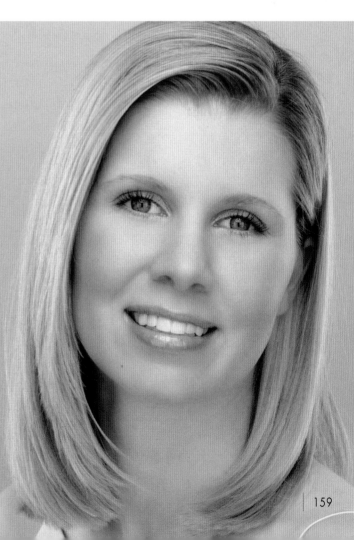

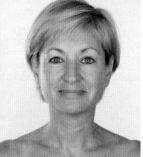

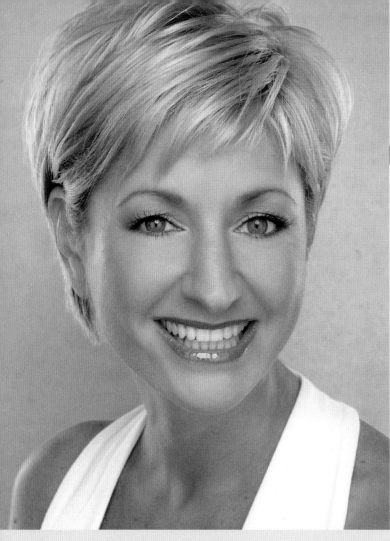

kathy helou

FACE SHAPE: square
EYE SHAPE: hooded
SHADOWS: Highlight: shimmer flesh
               Midtone: matte taupe
               Contour: shimmer golden brown
OBJECTIVE: To give the illusion of a more oval-shaped
face. To minimize the hooded appearance of her eyelids
making the eyes appear more open and alive.
APPLICATION: Contoured hairline and jaw to soften the
"four corners" of the face. Layered midtone and contour
colors on hooded areas of the eyelids. The layering of
color helps the end result appear more subtle and natural.

jordan helou

FACE SHAPE: square
EYE SHAPE: basic
SHADOWS: Highlight: shimmer beige
               Midtone: matte taupe
               Contour: shimmer golden brown
OBJECTIVE: To give the illusion of a more oval-shaped
               face. To subtly define her features.
APPLICATION: Contoured hairline and jaw to soften the
"four corners" of the face. Highlighted down the center
of the forehead, nose, and tip of the chin. Highlighted lids
and browbones, then defined eyes at lash line and in the
crease. Finished with glossy lips.

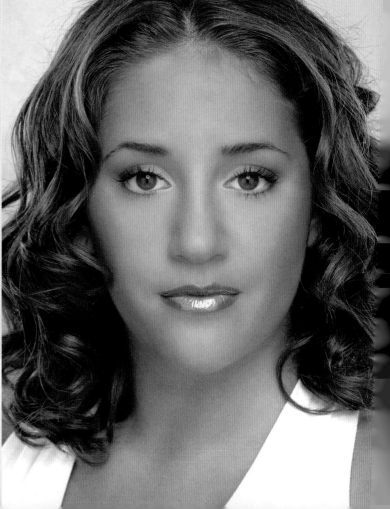

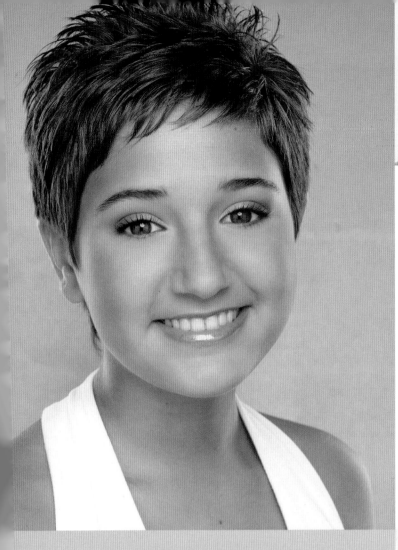

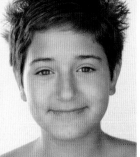

sidney helou

FACE SHAPE: square
EYE SHAPE: basic
SHADOWS: Highlight: shimmer beige
               Midtone: matte taupe
               Contour: shimmer golden brown
OBJECTIVE: To give the illusion of a more oval-shaped face. To subtly define her features.
APPLICATION: Her skin was so amazing that I did not have to do much. Contoured hairline and jaw to soften the "four corners" of the face. Highlighted down the center of the forehead, nose, and tip of the chin. Highlighted her lids and browbones. Subtly defined her crease.

braden harris

FACE SHAPE: square
EYE SHAPE: hooded
SHADOWS: Highlight: shimmer flesh
               Midtone: matte taupe
               Contour: shimmer golden brown
OBJECTIVE: To give the illusion of a more oval-shaped face. To minimize the hooded appearance of her eyelids making the eyes appear more open and alive.
APPLICATION: Contoured hairline and jaw to soften the "four corners" of the face. Layered midtone and contour colors on hooded areas of the eyelids. The layering of color helps the end result appear more subtle and natural.

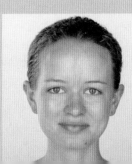

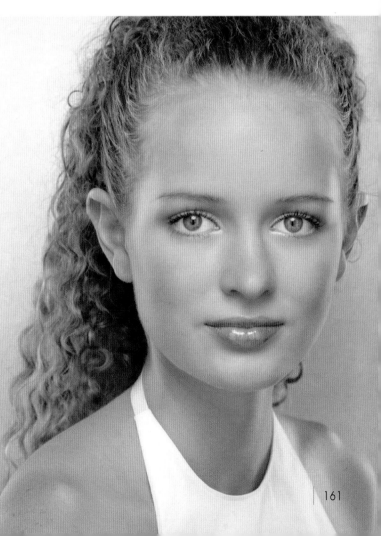

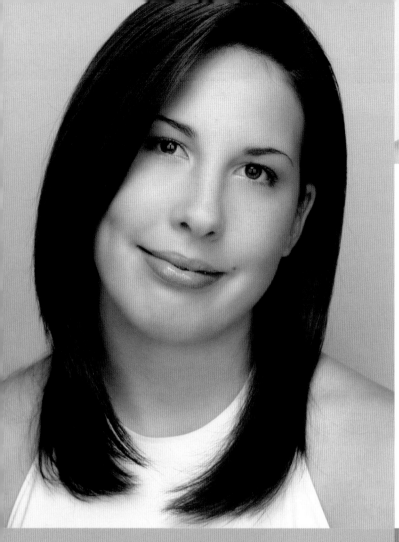

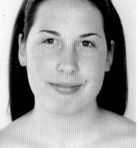

vanessa shasteen

FACE SHAPE: pear
EYE SHAPE: basic
SHADOWS: Highlight: shimmer flesh
Midtone: matte taupe
Contour: matte dark taupe
OBJECTIVE: To give the illusion of a more oval-shaped face and subtly define her features without making her look too mature.
APPLICATION: Contoured the jawline and cheeks to help minimize their width. Highlighted the center of the forehead to create the illusion of more width. Subtly defined the eyes at the lash line and glossed the lips to give her a fresh, young look.

stacy james

FACE SHAPE: long
EYE SHAPE: droopy
SHADOWS: Highlight: shimmer gold
Midtone: matte taupe
Contour: shimmer golden brown
OBJECTIVE: To make the outer corners of the eyes appear to turn up rather than down. To give the illusion of a more oval-shaped face.
APPLICATION: Made sure to begin all midtone and contour shadow application in slightly from the outside corner of the eye, making sure to blend up and in, not out and down. Made sure to put lots of color on the apples of the cheeks to visually shorten the length of face.

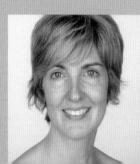

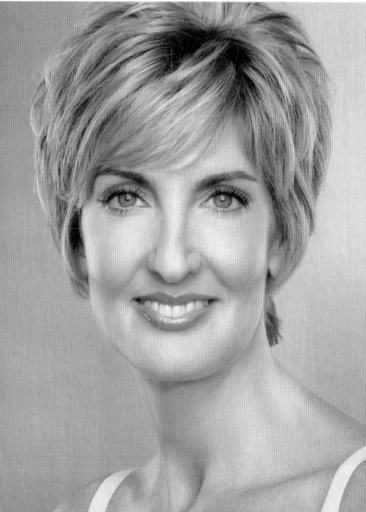

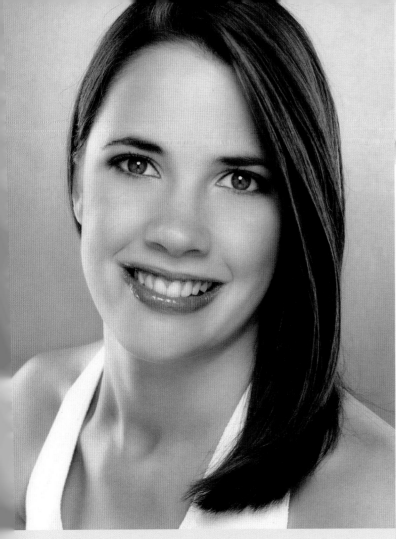

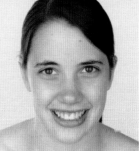

tess mullen

FACE SHAPE: oval
EYE SHAPE: basic
SHADOWS: Highlight: shimmer beige
Midtone: matte taupe
Contour: matte dark taupe
OBJECTIVE: To softly define the features and give her a polished, sophisticated look.
APPLICATION: With an oval-shaped face like Tess's, there was not a lot to do. Warmed up the skin with bronzer. Subtly defined the eyes by highlighting the lids and browbone, then softly defined the crease and lash line with soft colors.

stefanie cox

FACE SHAPE: square
EYE SHAPE: wide-set
SHADOWS: Highlight: shimmer beige
Midtone: matte taupe
Contour: matte dark brown
OBJECTIVE: To give the illusion of a more oval-shaped face and help the eyes appear closer together.
APPLICATION: Contoured the hairline and jaw to soften the "four corners" of the face. Highlighted down the center of the forehead, nose, and tip of the chin. Layered midtone color in the crease and on the inside hollow of the eyes to visually pull the eye placement closer together.

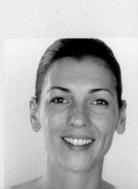

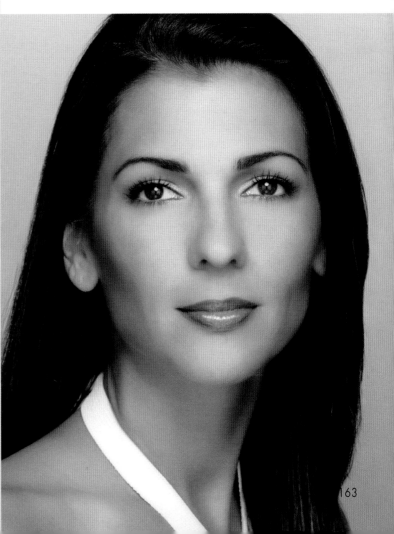

163

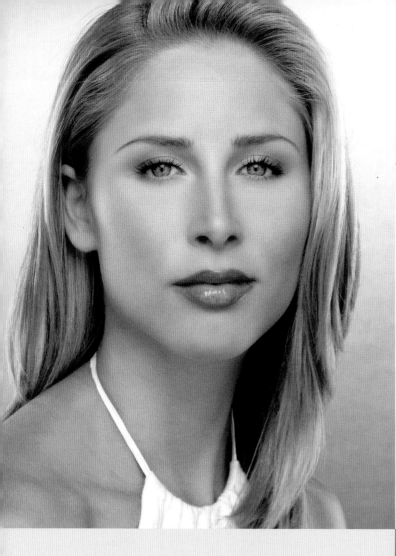

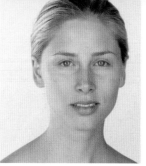

poppi monroe

FACE SHAPE: square
EYE SHAPE: basic
SHADOWS: Highlight: shimmer flesh
Midtone: matte taupe
Contour: shimmer golden brown
OBJECTIVE: To create the illusion of a more oval-shaped face and to subtly define her features.
APPLICATION: Contoured the hairline and jaw to soften the "four corners" of the face. Highlighted the center of the forehead, nose, and tip of the chin. Highlighted the lid and browbone to open up the eye. Defined the crease and lash line to give the eye more shape.

julianne

FACE SHAPE: square
EYE SHAPE: deep-set
SHADOWS: Highlight: shimmer beige
Midtone: matte taupe
Contour: shimmer golden brown
OBJECTIVE: To create the illusion of a more oval shaped face. To bring her eyes out and push brow bone back.
APPLICATION: Contoured the hairline and jaw to soften the "four corners" of the face. Highlighted the center of the forehead, nose, and tip of the chin. Highlighted lid only, to bring the eyes forward. Used midtone on browbone to push it away.

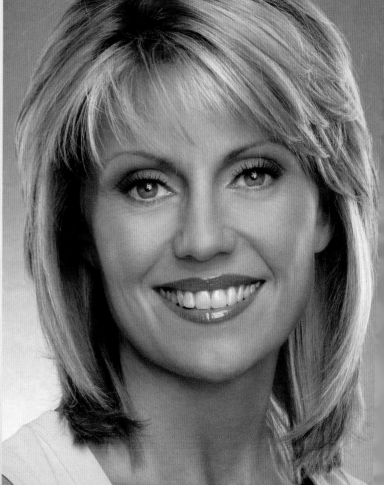

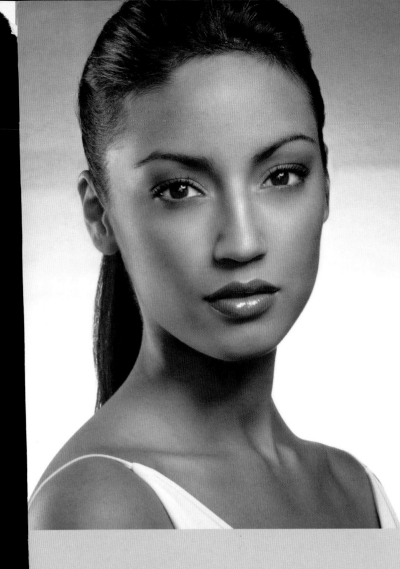

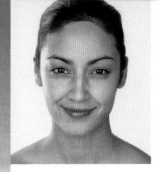

marisol

FACE SHAPE: oval
EYE SHAPE: basic
SHADOWS: Highlight: matte sand
              Midtone: matte caramel
              Contour: matte dark brown
OBJECTIVE: To define eyes and open them up. To give her skin a beautiful glow.
APPLICATION: Made sure to define really well at the lash line and curled her lashes to really bring her eyes out. Applied multiple layers of mascara one to lengthen, one to thicken. Used bronzer to give her skin a rich depth and followed it with a rich warm blush.

pam frank

FACE SHAPE: square
EYE SHAPE: hooded
SHADOWS: Highlight: shimmer flesh
              Midtone: matte taupe
              Contour: shimmer golden brown
OBJECTIVE: To give the illusion of a more oval-shaped face. To minimize the hooded appearance of her eyelids, making the eyes appear more open and alive.
APPLICATION: Contoured hairline and jaw to soften the "four corners" of the face. Highlighted forehead, under eyes on top of cheek bone and tip of chin. Layered midtone and contour colors on hooded areas of the eyelids. The layering of color helps the end result appear more subtle and natural.

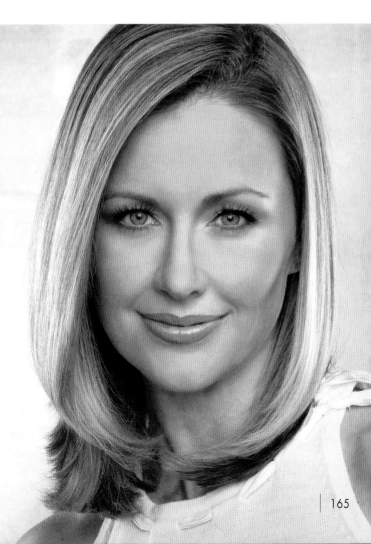

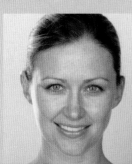

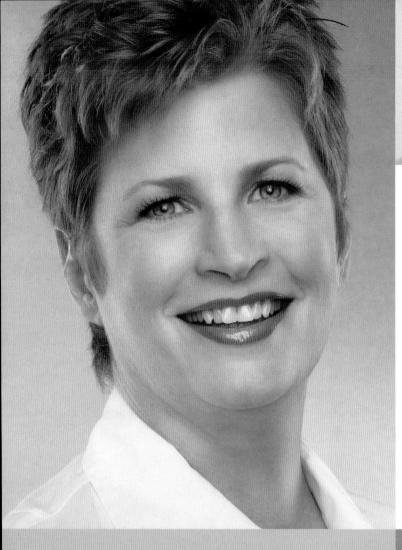

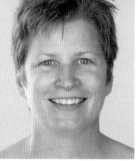

patty woodrich

FACE SHAPE:	pear
EYE SHAPE:	hooded
SHADOWS:	Highlight: shimmer flesh
	Midtone: matte taupe
	Contour: shimmer golden brown

OBJECTIVE: To create the illusion of a more oval-shaped face and to help her hooded eyelids recede.

APPLICATION: Contoured jawline and cheeks to help minimize their width. Highlighted the center of the forehead to create the illusion of more width. Layered midtone and contour colors on hooded areas. The layering of color helps the end result appear more subtle and natural.

debi moore

FACE SHAPE:	oval
EYE SHAPE:	deep-set
SHADOWS:	Highlight: shimmer beige
	Midtone: matte taupe
	Contour: shimmer golden brown

OBJECTIVE: To bring her eyes out and push browbone back. To give her skin a beautiful glow. Make her lips look fuller.

APPLICATION: Highlighted lids only, to bring the eyes forward. Used midtone on browbone to push it away. Used bronzer on cheeks and temples, ended by choosing a soft warm blush to give her a glow. Used lip enhancing technique to make them appear larger.

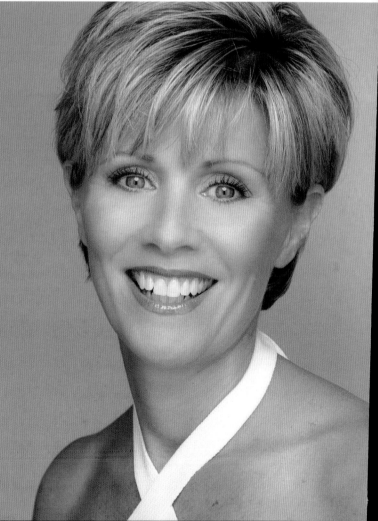

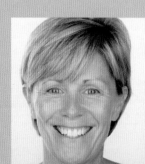

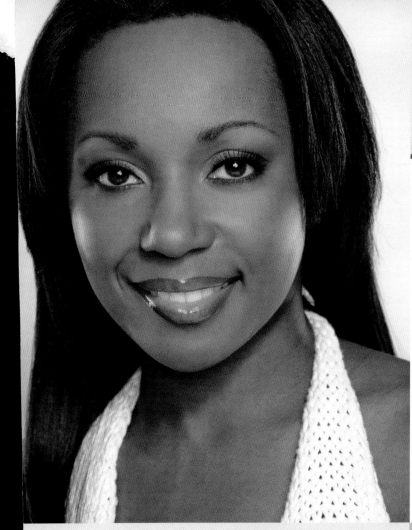

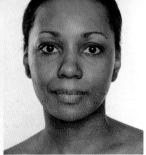

lori jones

FACE SHAPE: square
EYE SHAPE: basic
SHADOWS: Highlight: shimmer gold
Midtone: matte mahogany
Contour: matte dark brown
OBJECTIVE: To give the illusion of a more oval-shaped face. To even out and brighten her skin tone.
APPLICATION: Contoured the hairline and jaw to soften the "four corners" of the face. Highlighted down the center of the forehead, nose, and tip of the chin. Highlighted the lid and browbone. To even out the skin tone, used multiple shades of foundation then brightened the skin with a golden-orange face powder on all highlight areas of the face.

elaine moock

FACE SHAPE: square
EYE SHAPE: hooded
SHADOWS: Highlight: shimmer flesh
Midtone: matte taupe
Contour: shimmer golden brown
OBJECTIVE: To give the illusion of a more oval-shaped face. To minimize the hooded appearance of her eyelids making the eyes appear more open and alive.
APPLICATION: Contoured hairline and jaw to soften the "four corners" of the face. Layered midtone and contour colors on hooded areas of the eyelid. The layering of color helps the end result appear more subtle and natural.

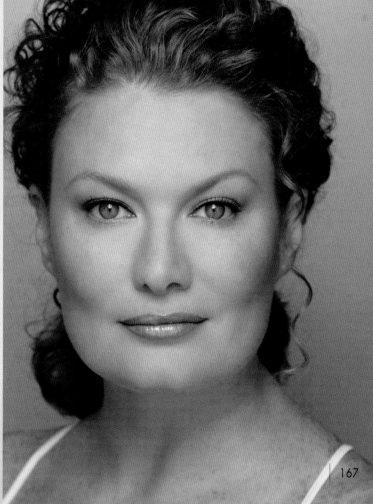

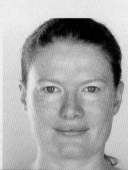

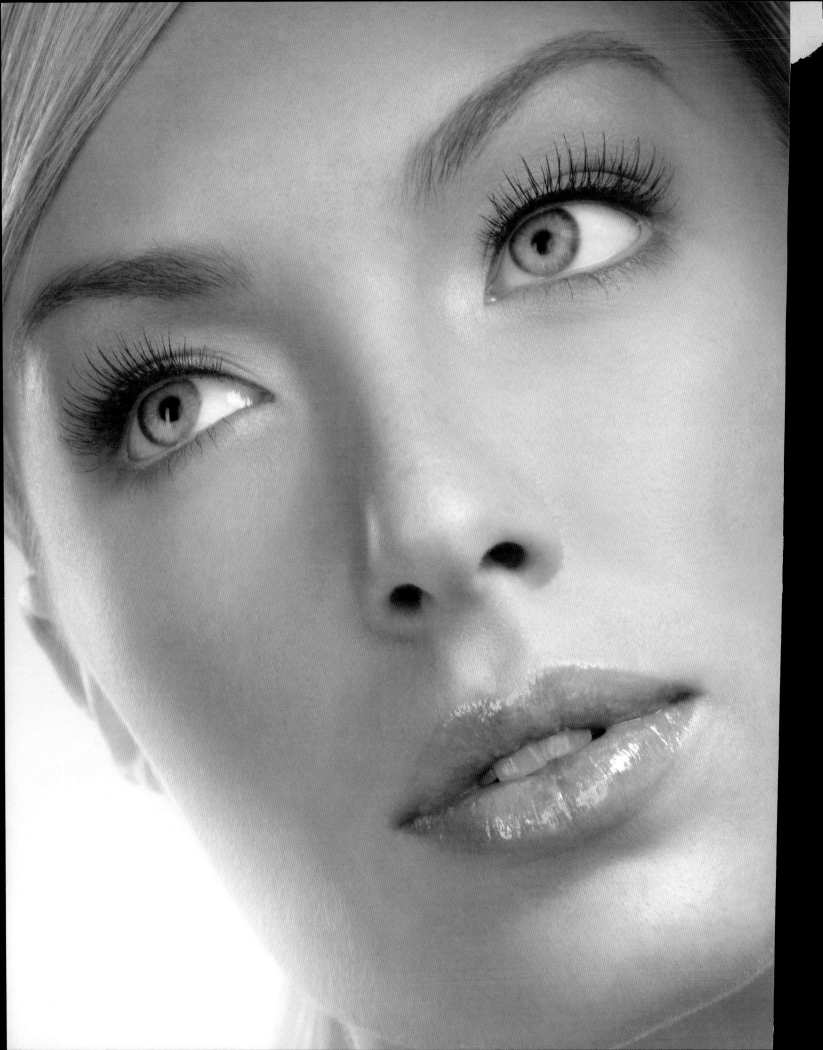

12

models
need makeup too

Everyone thinks that models are perfect, but even though they are
pretty darn close to it, even they can benefit from a little makeup.
In this chapter, I have taken models that I feel are some of the most
beautiful and have shown you that even though they are truly
beautiful without makeup, with it they are drop-dead beautiful.
(I just think it's nice to know that even models wake up looking like
you!) So enjoy seeing their transformations and know that you are
just as beautiful as they are.

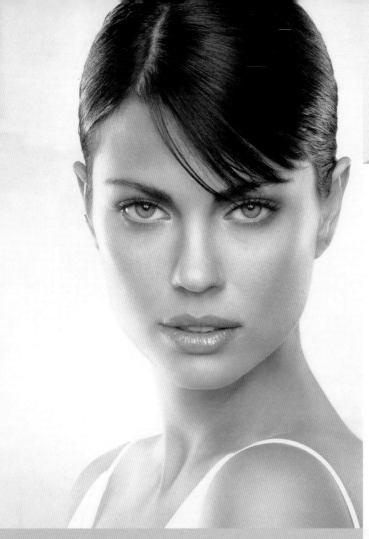

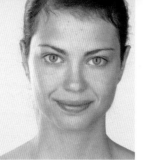

fabiana

FACE SHAPE: square
EYE SHAPE: basic
SHADOWS: Highlight: shimmer beige
               Midtone: matte taupe
               Contour: shimmer golden brown
OBJECTIVE: To give her face the illusion of being a
bit more oval. Bring out those beautiful eyes.
APPLICATION: Bronzed and contour the "four corners"
of the face. Highlighted the forehead, underneath the
eyes on top of the cheek bone, and the chin. Applied
deepest shade liberally along lash line to bring out eye
color and define.

cynthia

FACE SHAPE: square
EYE SHAPE: basic
SHADOWS: Highlight: shimmer white gold
               Midtone: matte mahogany
               Contour: shimmer purple
OBJECTIVE: To give the illusion of a more oval-shaped
face. To even out skin tone and brighten areas to add
life to the face.
APPLICATION: Using multiple shades of foundation,
evened out the slight skin discoloration. The main goal
was to brighten her face, which was achieved by using
a golden orange face powder to highlight areas.
Contoured hairline and jaw to soften the "four corners"
of the face.

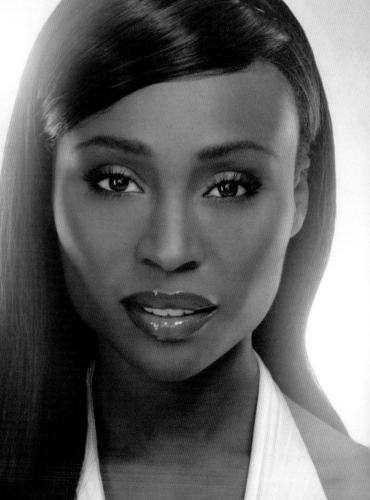

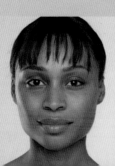

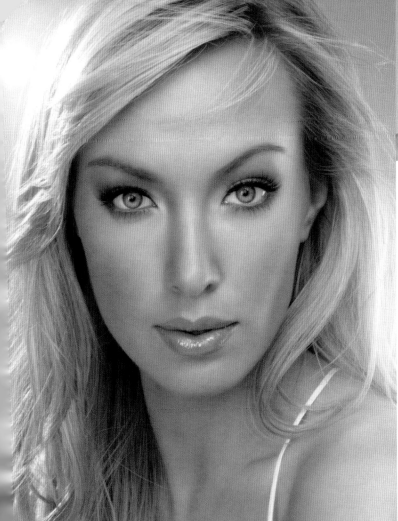

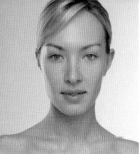

kate

FACE SHAPE: oval
EYE SHAPE: basic
SHADOWS: Highlight: shimmer flesh
Midtone: matte taupe
Contour: matte caramel
OBJECTIVE: To draw all the attention to those unbeliev-able blue eyes. Give the skin a glow.
APPLICATION: Chose all shades of eyeshadow that had really strong warm undertones so that all the attention would be on the blue in the eyes. Did not have to use dark shadows to define, because the warm undertone really intensified the blue. Applied bronzer to cheeks and temples, giving the skin an amazing glow. Also soft warm lips helped pop the blue in the eyes as well.

nonna

FACE SHAPE: oval
EYE SHAPE: basic
SHADOWS: Highlight: shimmer gold
Midtone: matte taupe
Contour: matte dark taupe
OBJECTIVE: To really bring out her eyes and give skin a glow.
APPLICATION: Curled then applied many, many coats of mascara to lashes to really define her eyes without a lot of dark eyeshadow. Made sure to apply mascara vertically and horizontally so her lashes would be thick and long. Used very soft lip color so the attention is drawn to the eyes. Used bronzer on cheeks and temples to give the face a glow.

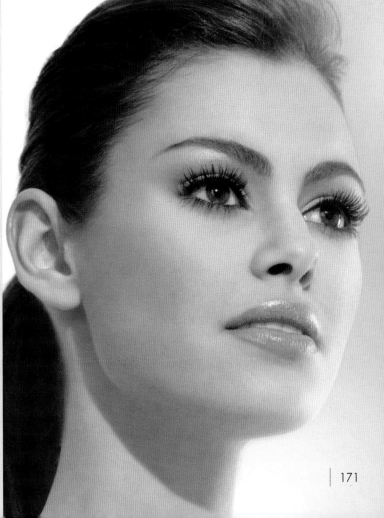

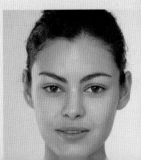

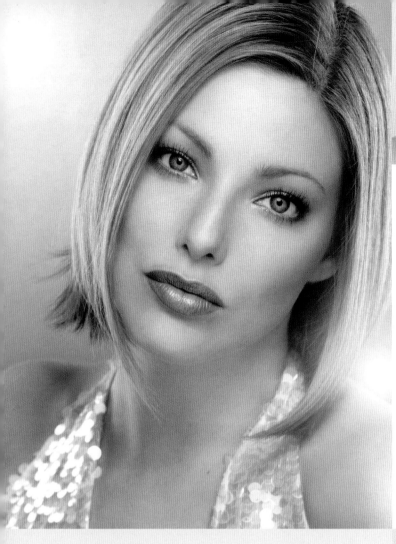

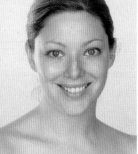

kate

FACE SHAPE: oval
EYE SHAPE: hooded
SHADOWS: Highlight: shimmer flesh
               Midtone: matte taupe
               Contour: shimmer golden brown
OBJECTIVE: To minimize the hooded appearance of her eyelids, making the eyes appear more open and alive. Give skin a beautiful glow.
APPLICATION: Layered midtone and contour colors on hooded areas of the eyelids. The layering of color helps the end result appear more subtle and natural. Curled lashes really well, helping to open the eyes. Used bronzer on cheeks and temples to give a glow, followed by warm colorful blush.

lauren

FACE SHAPE: square
EYE SHAPE: basic
SHADOWS: Highlight: shimmer gold
               Midtone: matte taupe
               Contour: shimmer copper
OBJECTIVE: To give her face the illusion of being a bit more oval. Bring out those beautiful brown eyes.
APPLICATION: Bronzed and contour the "four corners" of the face. Highlighted the forehead, underneath the eyes, on top of the cheek bone, and the chin. Applied deepest shade liberally along lash line to define the shape really well.

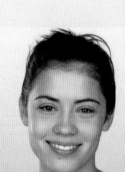

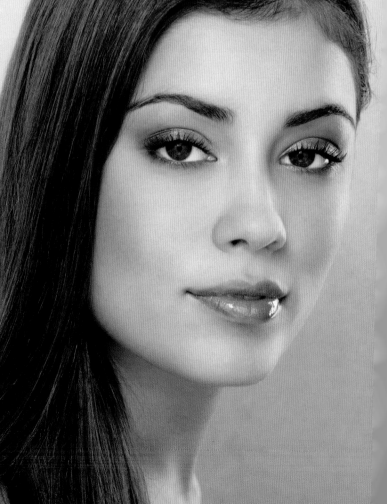

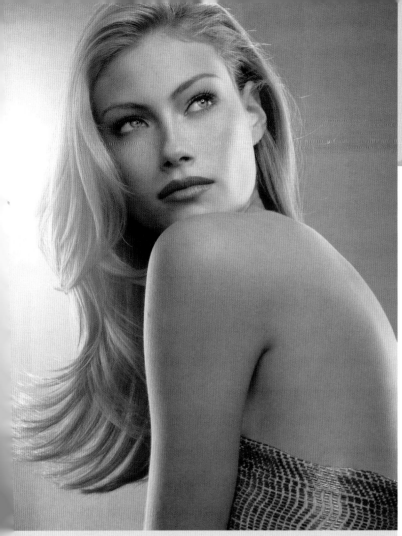

alyssa

FACE SHAPE: square
EYE SHAPE: basic
SHADOWS: Highlight: matte flesh
Midtone: matte taupe
Contour: matte brown
OBJECTIVE: To give her face the illusion of being a bit more oval. To give skin color and depth
APPLICATION: Bronzed and contour the "four corners" of the face. Highlighted the forehead, underneath the eyes on top of the cheek bone and the chin. Gave her colorful blush on the apples of her cheeks for more depth and life to skin.

glenna

FACE SHAPE: oval
EYE SHAPE: basic
SHADOWS: Highlight: shimmer flesh
Midtone: matte taupe
Contour: shimmer purple
OBJECTIVE: To give her skin some color and a glow. Draw attention to her eyes.
APPLICATION: Warmed up her skin by using one shade darker foundation followed by bronzer on her cheeks and temples, to give her skin more color but look natural. Used lots of color on her eyes to grab attention.

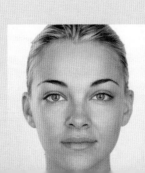

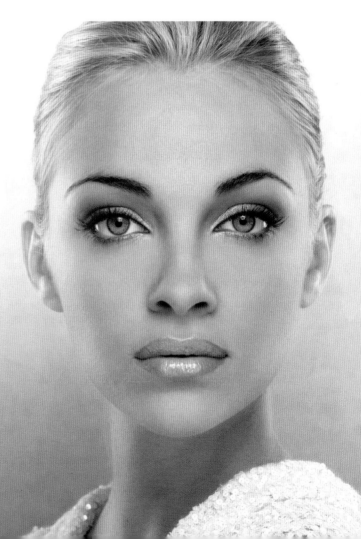

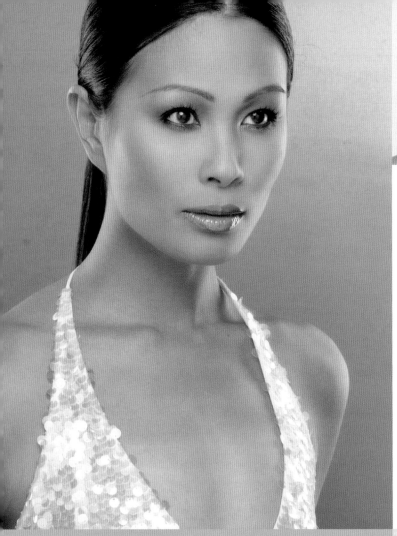

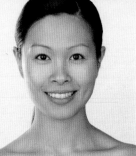

eleanor

FACE SHAPE: oval
EYE SHAPE: hooded
SHADOWS: Highlight: shimmer beige
              Midtone: matte dark taupe
              Contour: shimmer green brown
OBJECTIVE: To minimize the hooded appearance
of the eyelids, causing her eyes to appear more open
and alive.
APPLICATION: Applied midtone and contour color to
the hooded area of the lids to help them recede and open
up the eyes. Subtly layered color, starting with one layer
of midtone then following with additional layers to help
the hooded area appear to recede naturally.

sylvia

FACE SHAPE: round
EYE SHAPE: hooded
SHADOWS: Highlight: shimmer beige
              Midtone: matte taupe
              Contour: matte dark brown
OBJECTIVE: To minimize the hooded appearance
of the eyelids, causing her eyes to appear more open
and alive. To give the illusion of a more oval-shaped face.
APPLICATION: Applied midtone and contour color to
the hooded area of the lids to help them recede and open
up the eyes. Subtly layered color, starting with one layer
of midtone then following with additional layers, to help
the hooded area appear to recede naturally. Contoured
all along outer edge of face to minimize the width.
Highlighted forehead, underneath the eyes, on top
of cheek bones, and tip of chin.

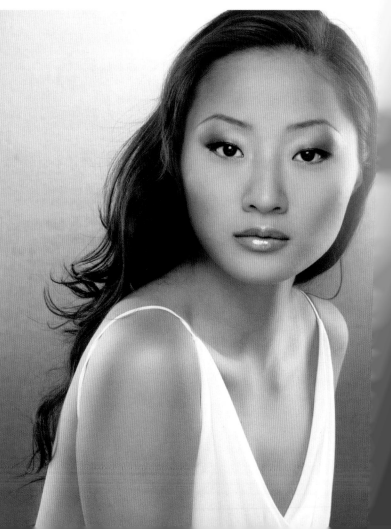

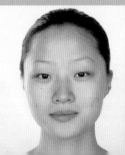

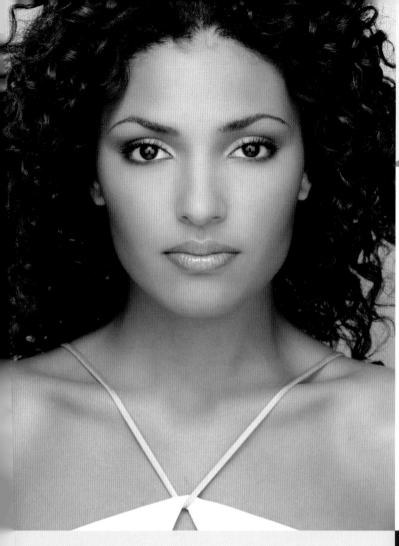

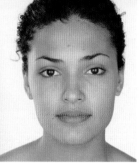

carol

FACE SHAPE: square
EYE SHAPE: basic
SHADOWS: Highlight: shimmer gold
Midtone: matte caramel
Contour: shimmer copper
OBJECTIVE: To give the illusion of a more oval- shaped face. To bring out her naturally beautiful skin tone.
APPLICATION: Bronzed and contour the "four corners" of the face. Highlighted the forehead, underneath the eyes, on top of the cheek bone, and the chin. Chose shades of eyeshadow, blush, and lipstick that all work to complement her bronze skin tone, giving her a natural glow.

alischia

FACE SHAPE: square
EYE SHAPE: basic
SHADOWS: Highlight: shimmer gold
Midtone: matte mahogany
Contour: matte black
OBJECTIVE: To give the illusion of a more oval-shaped face. To even out skin tone and brighten areas to add life to the face.
APPLICATION: Using multiple shades of foundation, evened out the slight skin discoloration. The main goal was to brighten her face, which was achieved by using a golden orange face powder to highlight areas. Contoured hairline and jaw to soften the "four corners" of the face.

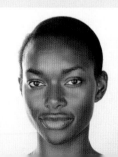

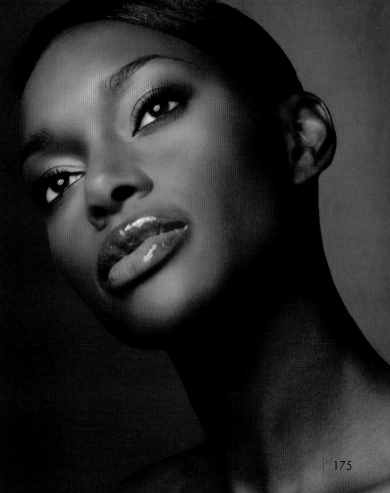

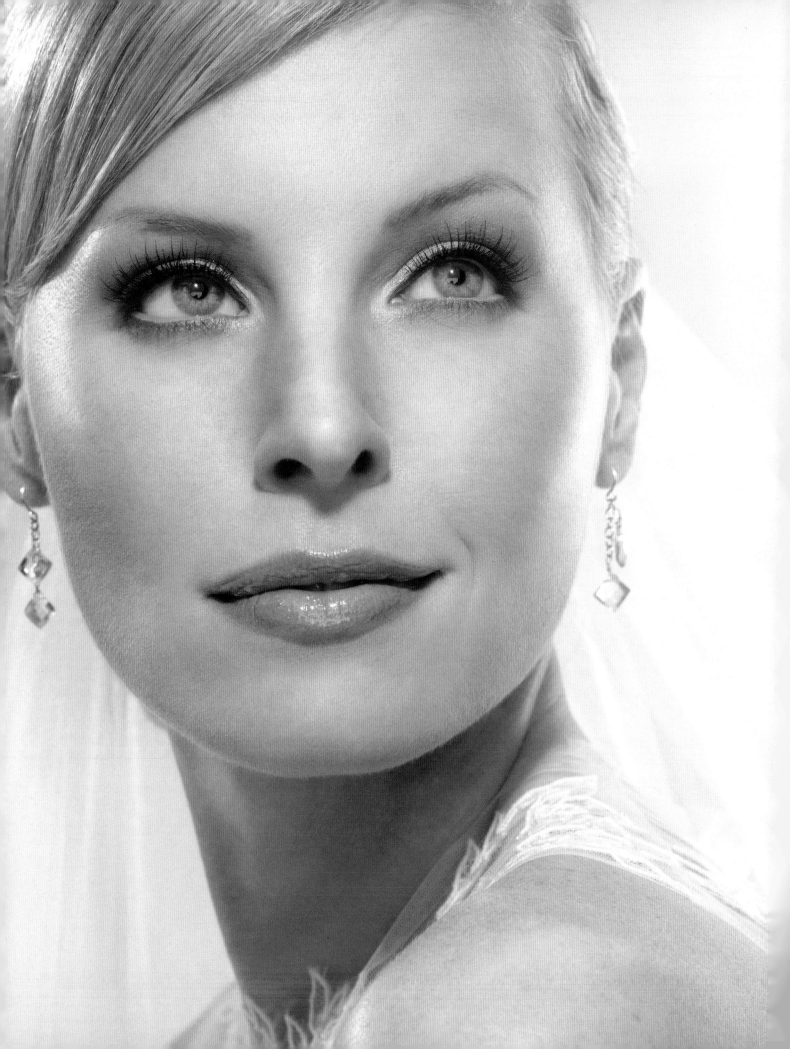

part four wedding perfection

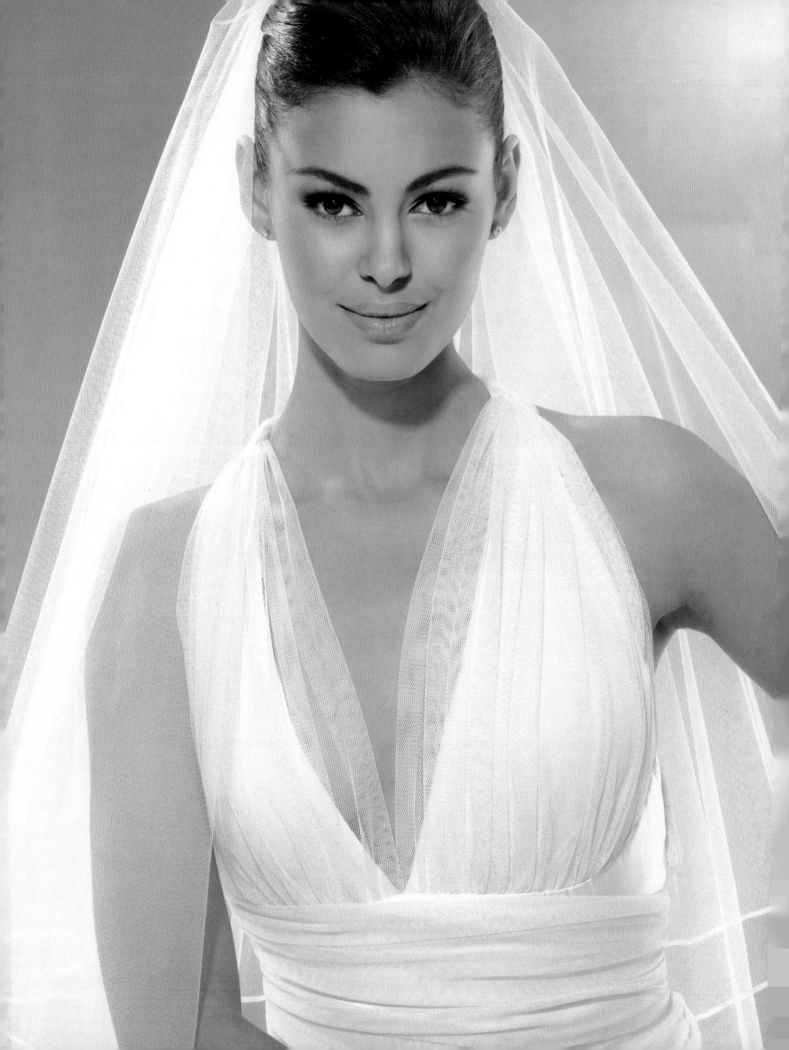

introduction
to bridal beauty

Your wedding day is so special and exciting. You are about to marry the person that you love and dream of spending forever with. I want to help you make it the most special day of your life. I have had the pleasure of helping some of the most beautiful women celebrate their wedding day. I count them among the most beautiful not because they were fashion models or famous actresses (although I have made up my share of those), but because they radiated a glow of love and excitement for the future.

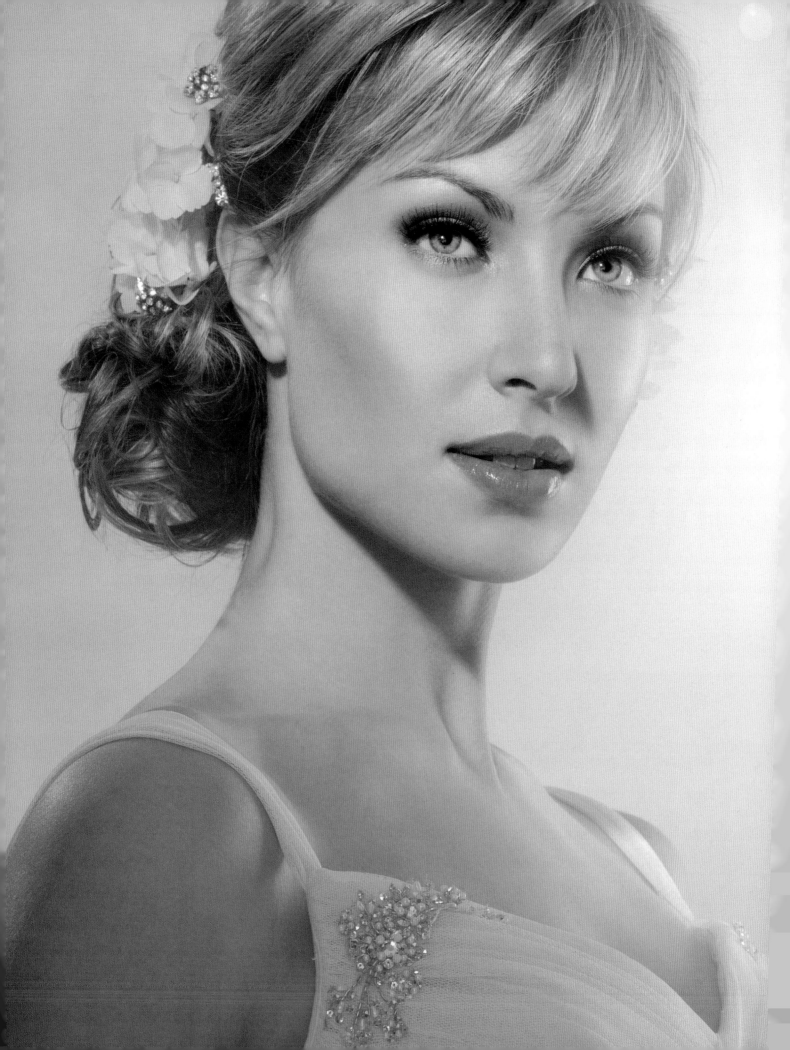

taking your time

When preparing for a wedding, most women spend weeks—even months—choosing the right dress. Then they'll spend weeks trying to find the perfect shoes. And then there's the time spent selecting the wardrobe for the entire bridal party. Many times, the anticipation leading up to the wedding is as much fun as the event itself.

I know you would not *dream* of waiting until the last minute to find the perfect wedding dress. Yet that's exactly what many women do when it comes to planning their makeup for the wedding and reception!

I want to make sure you're not one of them. You have to be prepared and ready for your day. It's important to find the perfect look ahead of time. You do not have to necessarily try something completely new, but you should fine-tune your look, and practice applying your makeup. The wonderful thing about makeup is that it will wash off, so feel free to play! If you don't get the look you want, you can always start over.

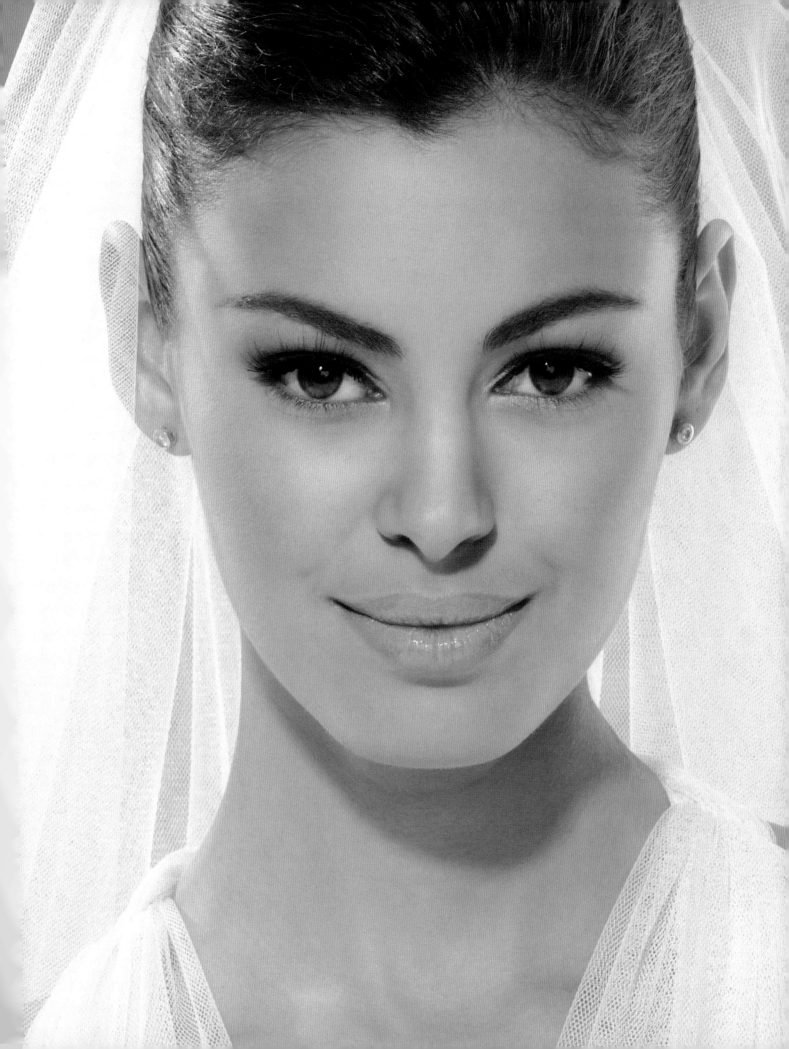

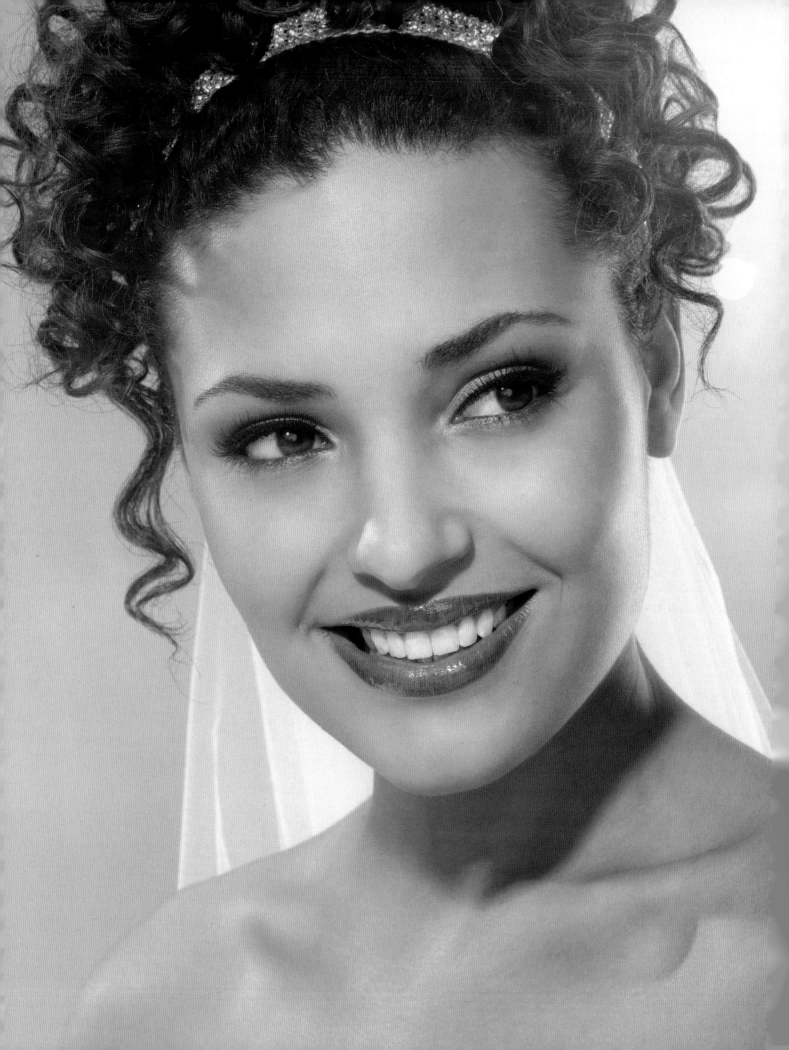

bridal beauty

I believe that choosing the look of your wedding day makeup is as important as choosing your gown. Yet so many women spend months looking for the perfect dress and thirty seconds deciding on the makeup look for their special day. Your look will be captured in photos forever, so it's important to put on your best face with no mistakes. After all, you are the very center of attention on your wedding day. Why leave your look to chance?

I will help you decide what kind of bride you want to be: a classic beauty, a glamour gal, or a sophisticated bride. With a little planning, practice, and advice, you and your entire bridal party can look picture-perfect on your wedding day.

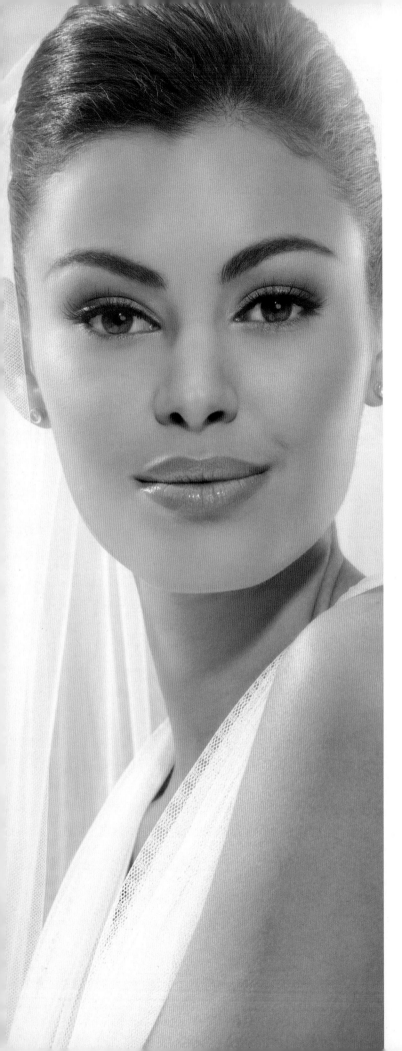

classic vs. trendy

The most important advice I can give you is this: Don't try a new look on the day of your wedding. Try new looks, maybe even several new looks, before your special day. This gives you a chance to see how all the looks appear before the day and to choose the one you really love.

Stay away from extreme makeup trends and go for a slightly more classic look that enhances your best features. You can go with something very modern or nontraditional if you want. You could even wear a color other than white for your special day.

Ask yourself this question: If you or your children were to look back on your wedding portrait and all the other photos fifteen years from now, would you still think you look pretty? That's a good rule of thumb to follow to decide if the makeup and hair looks you're choosing will stand the test of time.

Just make sure that, on your wedding day, you still look like you. You don't want to change your whole look so that people don't recognize you. Trust me, you don't want to overdo it and pile on the makeup. It is important to look like yourself—just the most beautiful you possible.

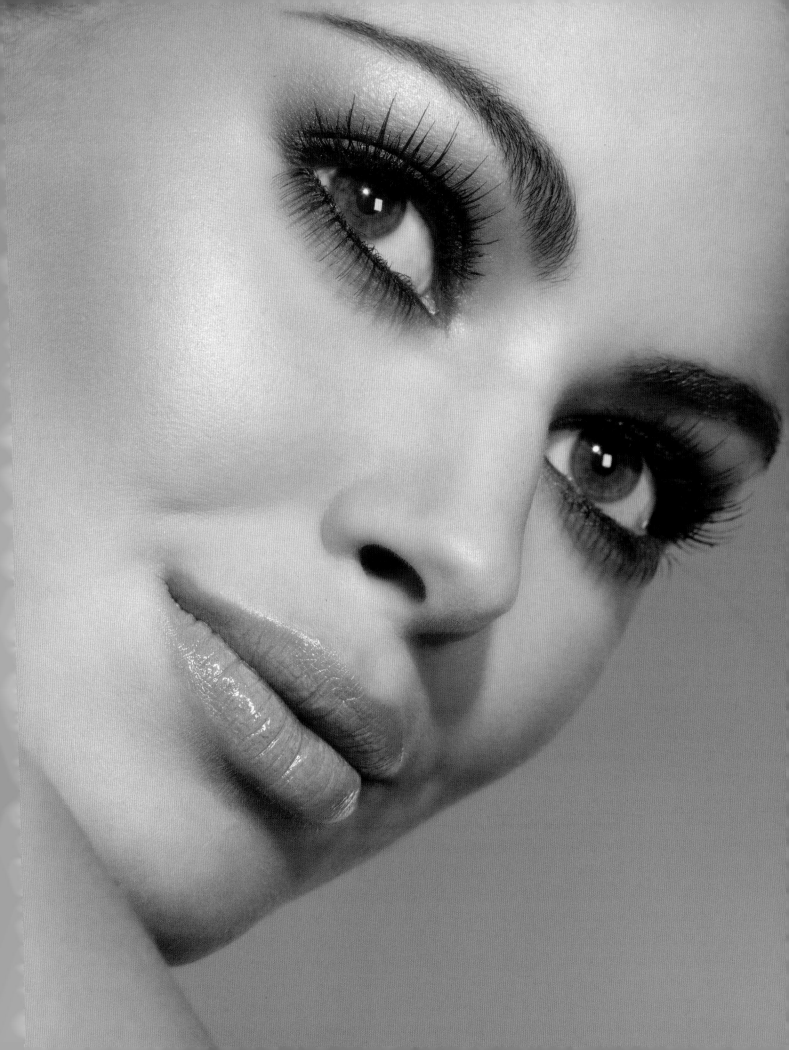

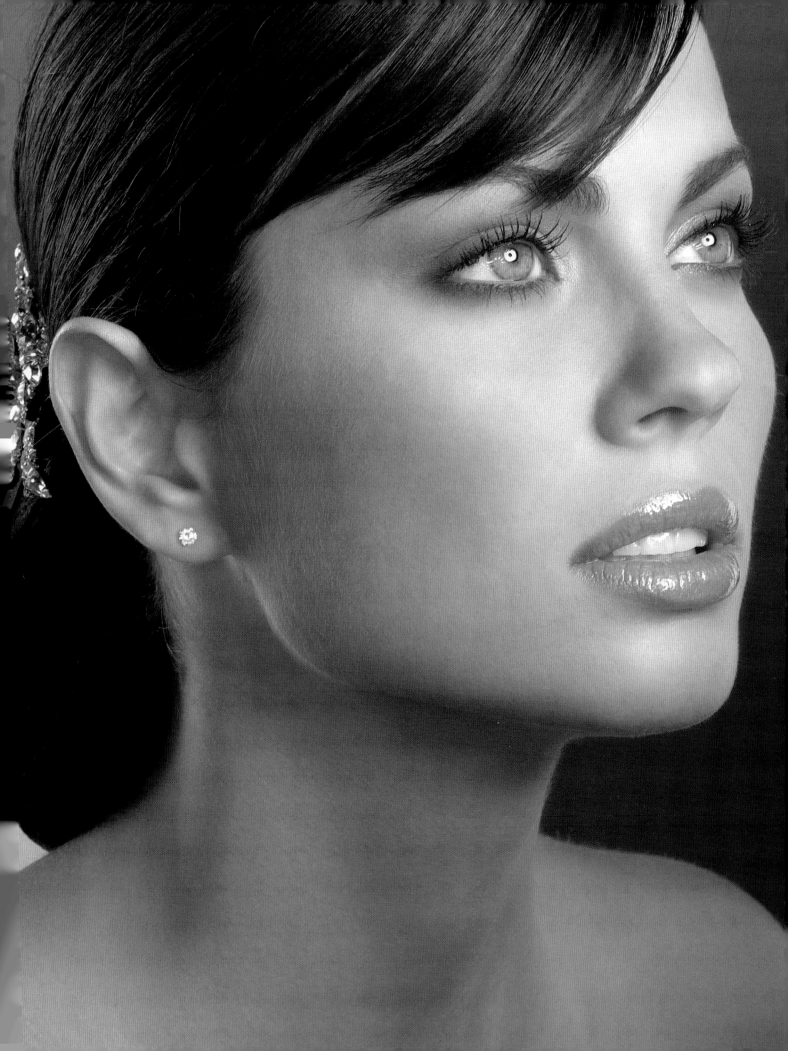

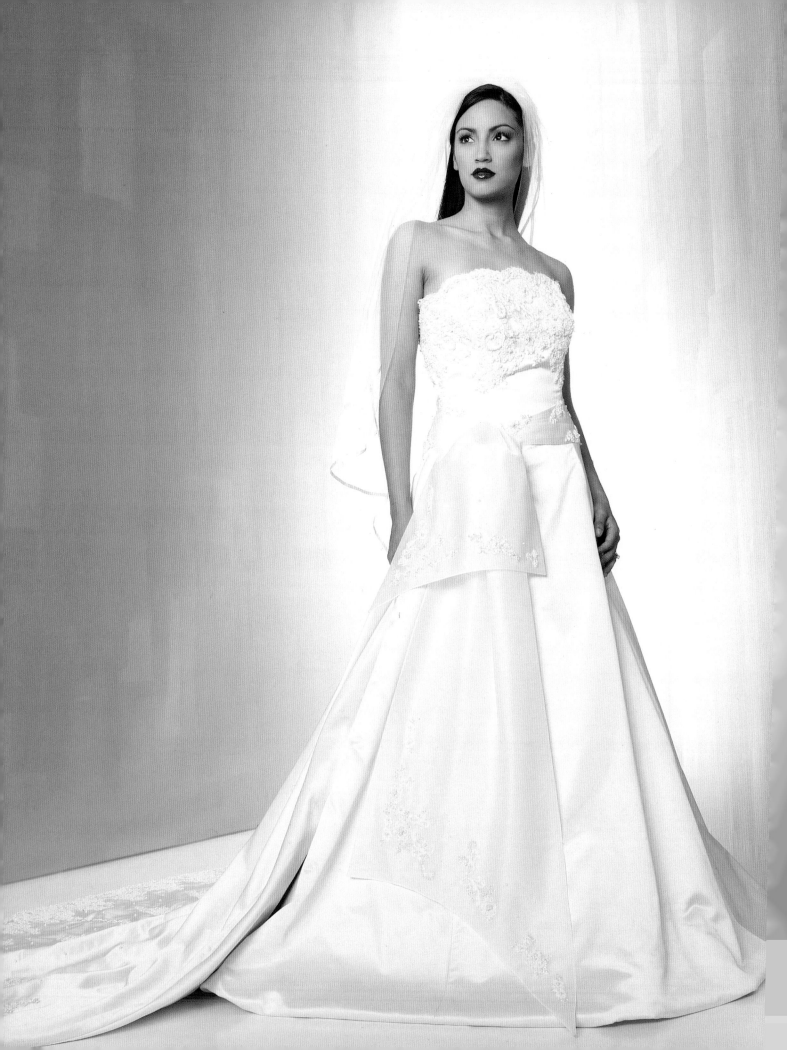

picture perfect

Here is another essential piece of advice: While you are trying new looks (*before* your wedding day, remember!), photograph them. I love to use a Polaroid camera, with its immediate gratification, but you could use a digital or disposable camera—whatever you have.

You will learn so much about what you have done and how each little change you make will photograph professionally. (I know that is hard to believe, but it's true.) Plus, it's fun! You could even make a party out of it: invite your bridesmaids over and have them do the same thing. I always take advantage of any reason to have a party!

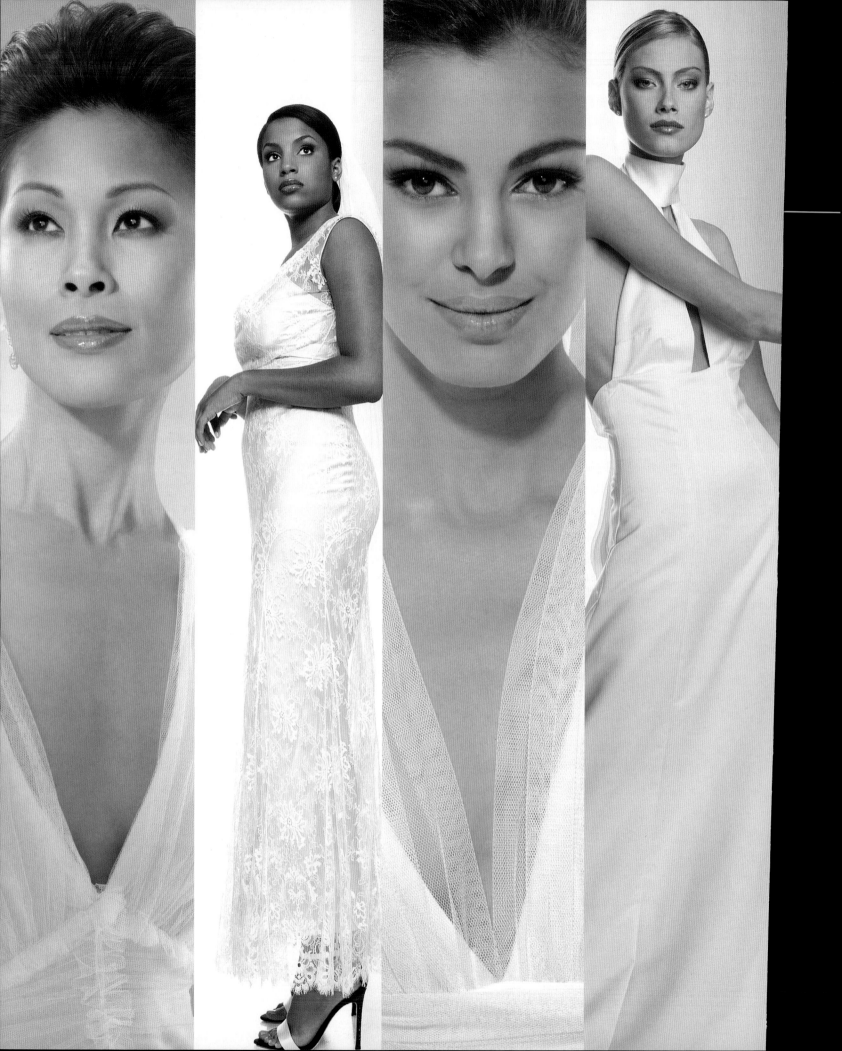

perfect **timing**

The time of day for your wedding will affect your makeup
choices. A more natural look for a morning wedding varies greatly
from the more dramatic look of an evening ceremony. The way
the sunlight changes throughout the day can influence the way your
makeup appears in photos. It can also affect the type of lighting
your photographer will choose when he or she photographs you.
I divide brides into four categories, based on the time of day
they're getting married: morning, midday, late afternoon, and
evening. With each time choice, there are certain details you'll
want to consider. Paying attention to these details can help you
get the look, and the wedding photos, of your dreams.

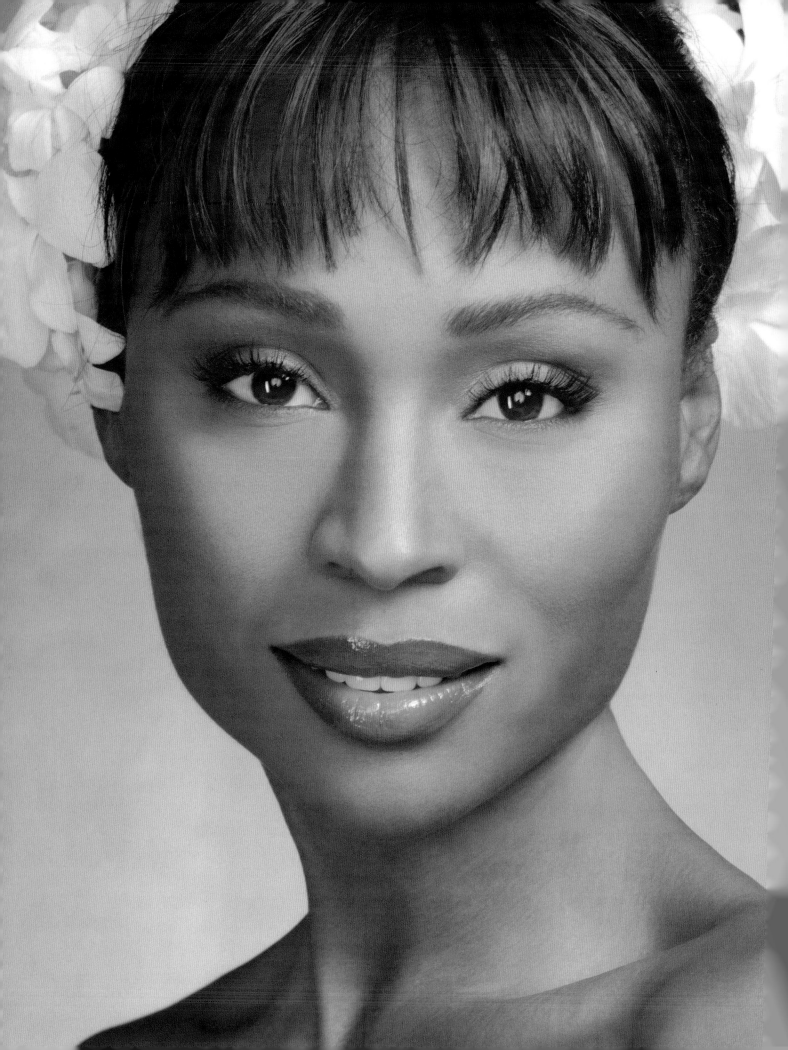

morning bride

If you're planning a morning wedding, your makeup look should appear soft and pretty to match the cool, soft morning light. Mornings are perfect for the natural girl, because it's the time of day when a bride should wear the least amount of makeup. I find that most brides who are getting married in the morning are having the event outside, or at least taking their photos and portraits outside. Even if they are getting married inside, the photographer will be taking advantage of the natural light coming through windows rather than a lot of artificial light for the photographs.

- Though a matte foundation is always perfect for photographs, a morning bride can choose to wear a foundation with a slight sheen or dewiness to it, because the light is so soft. Make sure that your skin is a nice, even tone.

- If your skin tends to break out, I would not choose this time of day for your wedding, because you are going to want to wear as little foundation and concealer as possible due to the softer natural light.

- Go light on the powder so your face retains its natural appearance. You want your skin to appear matte, but it does not take a lot of powder to achieve this. Heavy powder can appear artificial, especially in the morning light.

- Do not make bold eyeshadow color choices for your eyes if you are having a morning wedding. Choose warmer, soft shades that complement your eye color. This is the one time you will want to wear less eyeshadow, because the lighting will accentuate any harsh colors or lack of blending.

- Make sure to define your eyes really well at the lashline to help them stand out. To learn how to get the most from your mascara for great definition, see page 135. Another option would be false eyelashes; turn to page 206 for simple, foolproof application instructions.

- If you choose to wear eyeliner (you do not have to wear any) make sure to keep it subtle and soft. You do not want anything too dark (no black) or too harsh (not too thick—keep it really close to the lashline) at this time of day.

- Lip color should always be soft and natural—nothing too bold at this time of day. If it is too bold, it will be all you see in the photos.

- Everything will photograph darker than it appears to the eye, because the light is so soft, so go with softer shade choices.

- Bridesmaids' dresses should be in a soft color, and bridesmaids should also wear softer makeup shades.

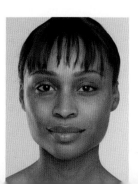

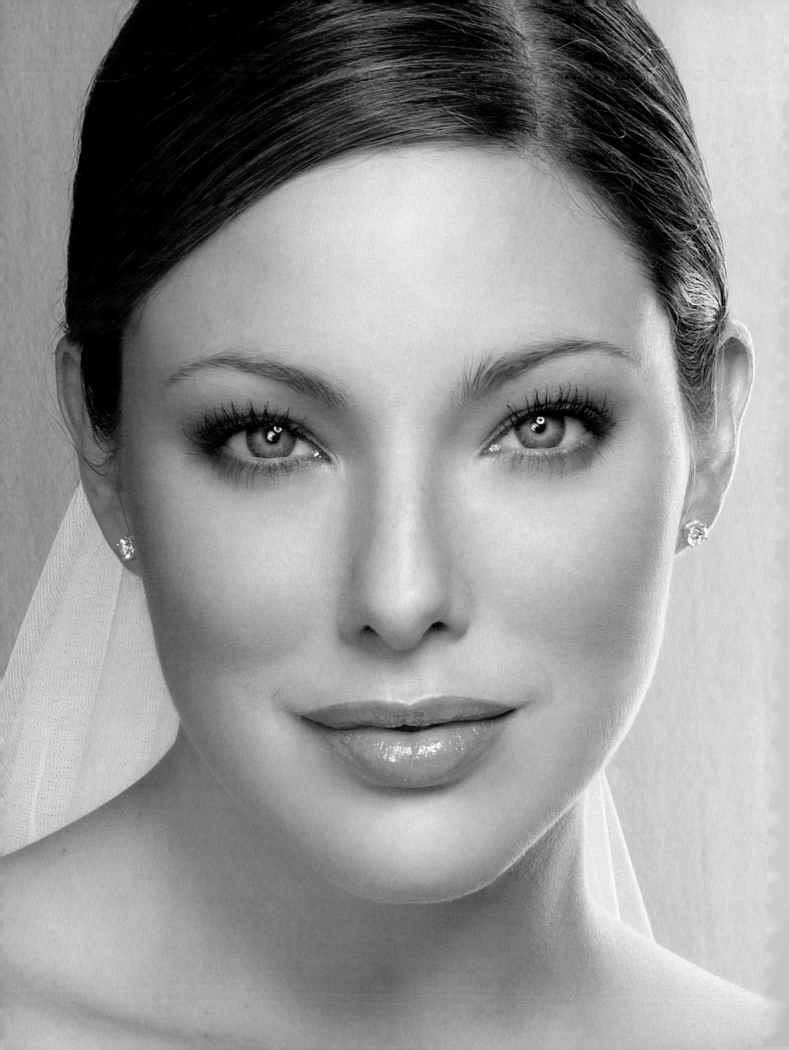

midday bride

If you're planning a wedding in the middle of the day, be aware that the midday sun can cast shadows on your face, which can make a difference if you're taking outdoor photos. This is the harshest light to be photographed in. Since natural light is directly above you at this time, you'll want to follow these steps to make sure you are "picture perfect."

- Do not wear foundation with a sheen or dewiness to it. If there is any sheen to the face, it will look too shiny and reflective in the photographs. This is a time when you will want to wear the least amount of foundation possible, because it will show the most. A lightweight foundation and a matte powder finish will photograph beautifully.

- Make sure your blush has a more matte finish, too. If it has too much shimmer, it will also look too shiny in the photos.

- A crème blush is a great choice for this time of day. It will absorb into your skin and look more natural. Keep in mind that crème blush does not work well on oily skin—stick with a powder blush if you fall into this category.

- Due to the midday lighting, if your eye makeup is too dark, your eyes will look like two dark holes in your photographs. Your highlight shade is the most important shadow choice at this time of day. Use a highlight with shimmer (not frost) to open up the eyes. The light-reflective particles in the shimmer will help prevent the "black hole effect." Make sure your midtone and/or contour shade has a matte finish—you never want to use three shades with shimmer, because the eye will look too shiny in the photographs. See page 129 for the perfect natural eyeshadow application process.

- If you want to wear eyeliner, keep it as close to the lashline as possible. If it is too thick, it could darken the lid more than you want, creating the dreaded "black hole effect."

- Long, beautiful lashes really help define your eyes without depending on heavy eyeliner. To learn how to get the most from your mascara, see page 135. False eyelashes would also be a perfect choice; turn to page 206 for foolproof application instructions.

- Since the sunlight grows stronger as midday approaches, every makeup line becomes more visible. Make sure to blend your foundation, blush, eyeshadow, and powder very well. At this time of day, there is no such thing as overblending.

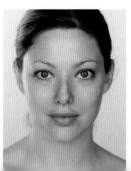

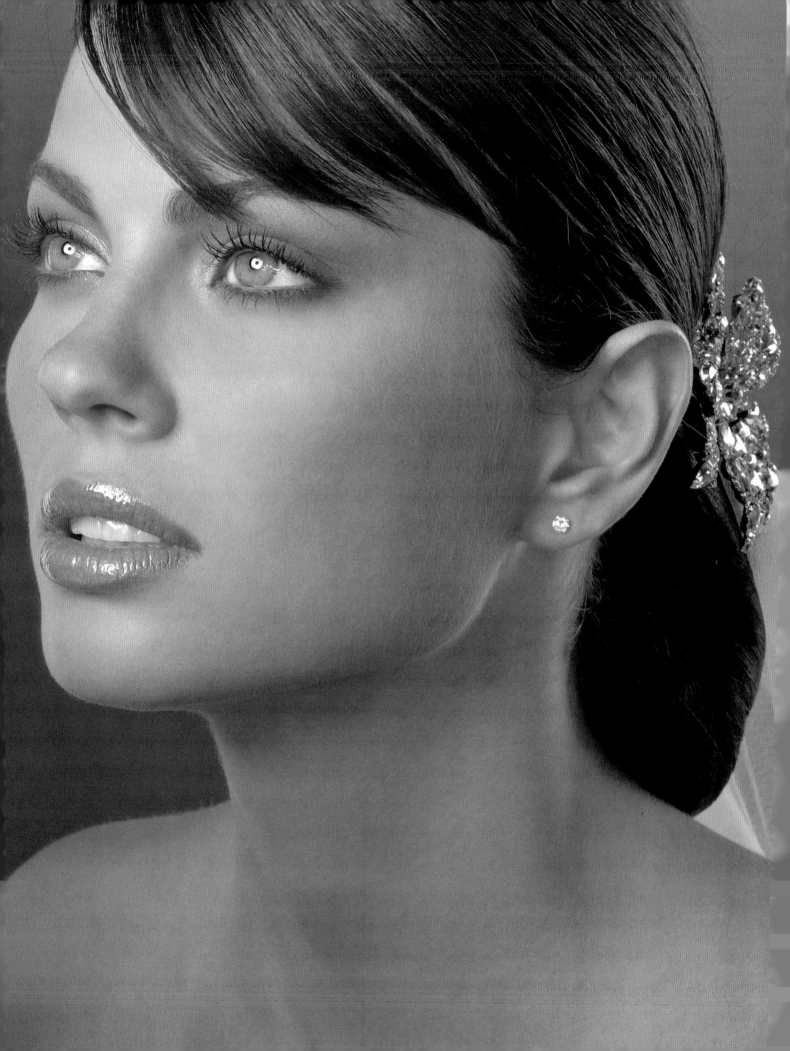

late-afternoon bride

The golden light of late afternoon is the most beautiful light you can be photographed in. Late afternoon is when the sun is starting to set in the sky, creating a beautiful warm glow. Since the light is so beautiful and forgiving, you can add a little more drama to your makeup look. The light is growing softer and warmer, so you can wear more eyeshadow and have more shade options.

- If your skin is less than perfect, late afternoon is a great time to get married. The light is softer and more forgiving, so you can use a little more foundation and concealer to cover your flaws, and your skin will still appear completely natural looking in photographs. Don't forget to powder— remember that matte skin always photographs better than shiny skin.

- As evening comes, your photographer will have to use a flash, so make sure you add color to your face. A flash shoots a bright burst of light at your face, which can make you appear washed out. Even if you do not normally wear blush on a daily basis, you need to wear at least a little color on your cheeks. I promise, you will not look or photograph like you belong on a street corner if you wear a soft bit of color on your cheeks! Another great way to prevent looking too

pale or washed out in your photos is to contour your face and add a warm glow with bronzing powder. To learn how to contour or "sculpt" your face, see page 83.

- It's fine for your blush to have shimmer in it, because it will look beautiful in this light, though it is also perfectly fine if you want to use a shade that is matte.

- You can make richer color choices because of the forgiving lighting. So feel free to apply more dramatic eyeshadow shades.

- A shimmery (not frosted) eyeshadow will look beautiful at this time of day, because it photographs well in all lighting. Just make sure that your midtone and/or contour shade has a matte finish. You never want to use three shades with shimmer, because the eye will look too shiny in photographs.

- Want to add a little more glamour? Try false eyelashes. This is the perfect time of day for this beauty trick, and lashes help define your eyes better than anything else you could do. Turn to page 206 to find out how to apply them. If you don't want to wear false lashes, then just make sure to layer your mascara to get the most definition you can. Turn to page 135 for layering techniques.

- Late-afternoon brides get the green light to wear a richer lip color, too. The light allows you to wear richer colors, since they won't show up in photos as too intense.

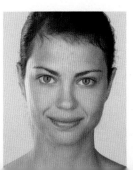

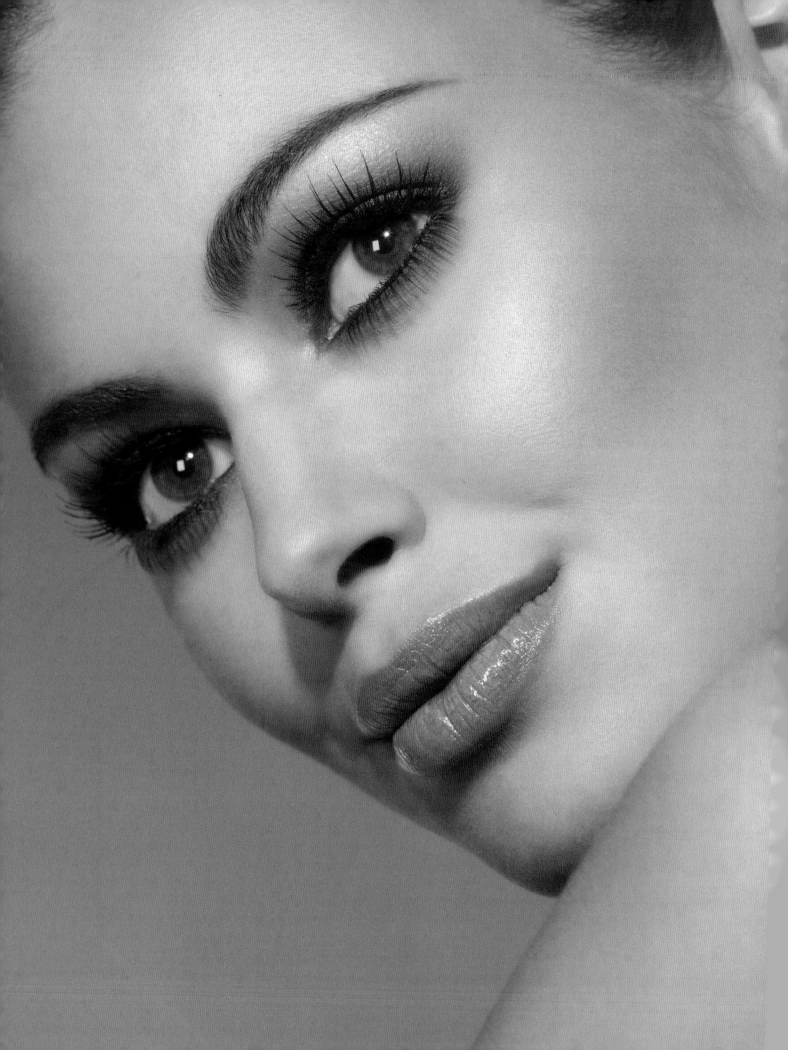

evening bride

If you love to glam it up, an evening wedding allows you to go for a more dramatic makeup look. You can play with color and wear more makeup than at any other time and still photograph beautifully. This is the time of day for the bride who wants to be a glamour queen. Remember that every photograph will be taken with a flash, which definitely makes a difference in your choices.

- If you have less than perfect skin, this is a great time for you. You can wear more foundation and powder and still look natural.

- Make sure to bronze generously to give your skin a glow. One thing that helps is "sculpting" your face, because it will add color so the flash will not wash your skin out, and it adds dimension. Dimension is important because the flash can also flatten everything out in a photograph. Turn to page 83 to learn how to use makeup to sculpt your face.

- Everything should be more defined—from your lips to your eyes to your cheekbones— because all photos will be taken with a flash, which, as I've mentioned, can wash you out. However, more defined does not mean darker. For instance, some women do not wear blush on a daily basis, but you need at least a little color in your cheek because of the flash. Make sure to give your lips a nice defined edge by lining; turn to page 142 for perfect application instructions. Also

for some women, especially natural blondes, even if you may not wear brow color on a daily basis, you may need a little so that your brows will show in the photos. Turn to page 127 for details on applying brow color.

- Shimmery eyeshadow will photograph well for evening, but you should wear absolutely no frosted shadows for this time of night (or any time for brides, in my opinion). Frosted eyeshadow will look too shiny in photos, especially when a flash is used! A shimmery shadow always looks soft and pretty. Just make sure that at least one of your three shades of shadow is matte. You never want all three shades to shimmer, because the eye will look too shiny in your photos.

- In my opinion, false eyelashes are a must for a nighttime wedding, because they help define the eyes really well. Just remember that every picture will be taken with a flash, and the more definition you have at your lashline, the better you will photograph. Turn to page 206 to find out how to apply false eyelashes. Not to worry if you do not want to wear false lashes, turn to page 135 to learn how to layer you mascara for maximum length and volume.

- If a smoky eye look is one you are interested in wearing, evening is a perfect time for this eyeshadow application technique. Learn how to apply it on page 221. Just make sure to wear a soft lip color if you're wearing a smoky eye.

- Make sure you have lip color and powder on at all times. You never know when the camera will flash!

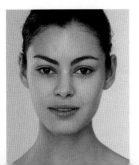

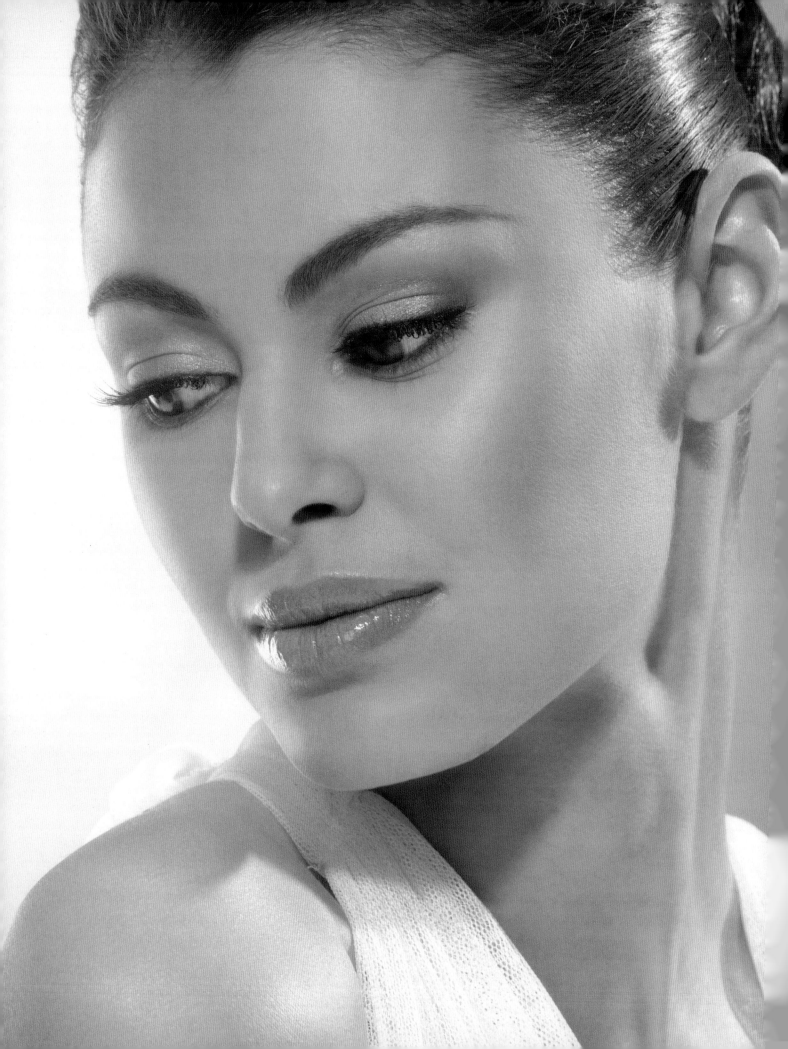

be a **pro**

I am going to share some pro tips that will make you look your best for you big day. I think that the key to your wedding day makeup is to apply it so the color lasts throughout the whole event. I want you to have to touch up as little as possible.

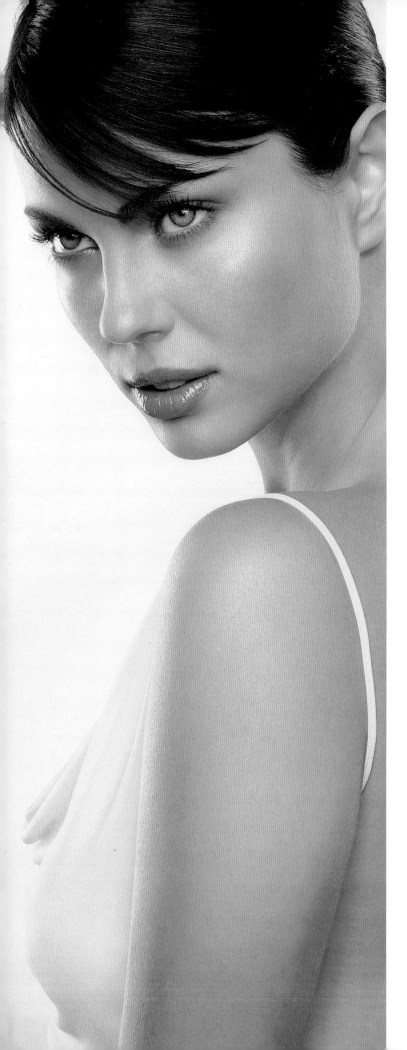

sunless tanning

Because some photography can wash out the skin, you may want to apply a self-tanning lotion to your face and body, starting a few weeks before the wedding to make sure you achieve the shade you want. Make sure you slowly build your color over time to make it appear more natural. Here is the best way to achieve smooth, even coverage when applying self-tanning lotion:

1. Exfoliate well.

2. Moisturize your skin to even out its porosity (your skin's ability to hold moisture).

3. For the body: Mix two parts self-tanner with one part moisturizer. Make sure to pour the self-tanner and moisturizer into a bowl and mix them completely together before you start. Do not try to mix the two in your hands as you apply it—the solution will not go on evenly. If you are very fair, you might want to mix one part self-tanning lotion with one part moisturizer to make it even more subtle.

4. For the face: Mix equal parts self-tanning lotion with moisturizer to dilute it, and apply it to your face over a period of days. If you are very fair, you might want to mix two parts moisturizer with one part self-tanning lotion to make it even more subtle. I recommend doing this gradually over a period of time instead of in one application, so your skin will get a slow build-up of color and appear more natural. If you have any dark spots, apply some petroleum jelly or a very thick moisturizer to the spot before you apply the self-tanning lotion; this will prevent the spot from taking color or darkening as the rest of your skin tans.

Bronzing powder is also a good choice. It can add warmth to your skin and give you a healthy, happy glow in your photographs. It is also much easier to apply, and you do not have to start weeks in advance. But bronzing powder is only good for adding color to your face. You do not want to try to bronze your whole body with a powder bronzer! It will just make a big mess by rubbing off on your dress.

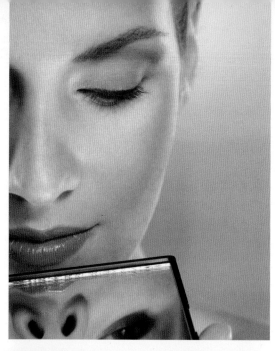

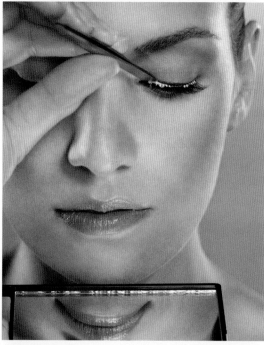

FALSE EYELASHES

Your wedding day is definitely the time to define your eyes. If you really want to draw attention to your eyes, you can always wear false eyelashes. I like using false eyelashes to define the eyes at the lashline instead of depending on heavy eyeliner and overly intense eyeshadow.

I know applying false eyelashes can seem intimidating, so here is an easy, foolproof way to apply false eyelashes. No matter what your make-up IQ is, this application technique will work for you and look natural. Just follow these easy steps to false eyelash perfection:

1. Curl your natural eyelashes.

2. Lay a mirror on the table or counter in front of you and look down.

3. Draw a thin line across your upper eyelid— right along your lashline—with an eyeliner pencil. This helps you know where to place the lash and helps conceal the lash band. This way, even if you do not get the false lash in place directly against your natural lashes, no one will know, because the liner will assure that no skin shows between your lashes and the false ones.

4. Trim the outside end of your false eyelashes to fit the width of your eyelid.

5. Apply eyelash glue to the false eyelashes. Allow the glue to dry for a minute so that it will get tacky (slightly sticky), then place the lash right on top of the eyeliner.

6. Once the glue has dried, apply one coat of mascara to blend your natural lashes with the false ones.

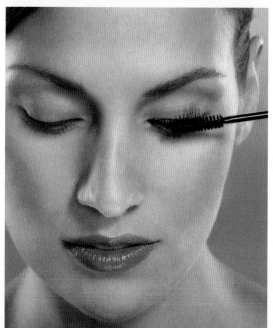

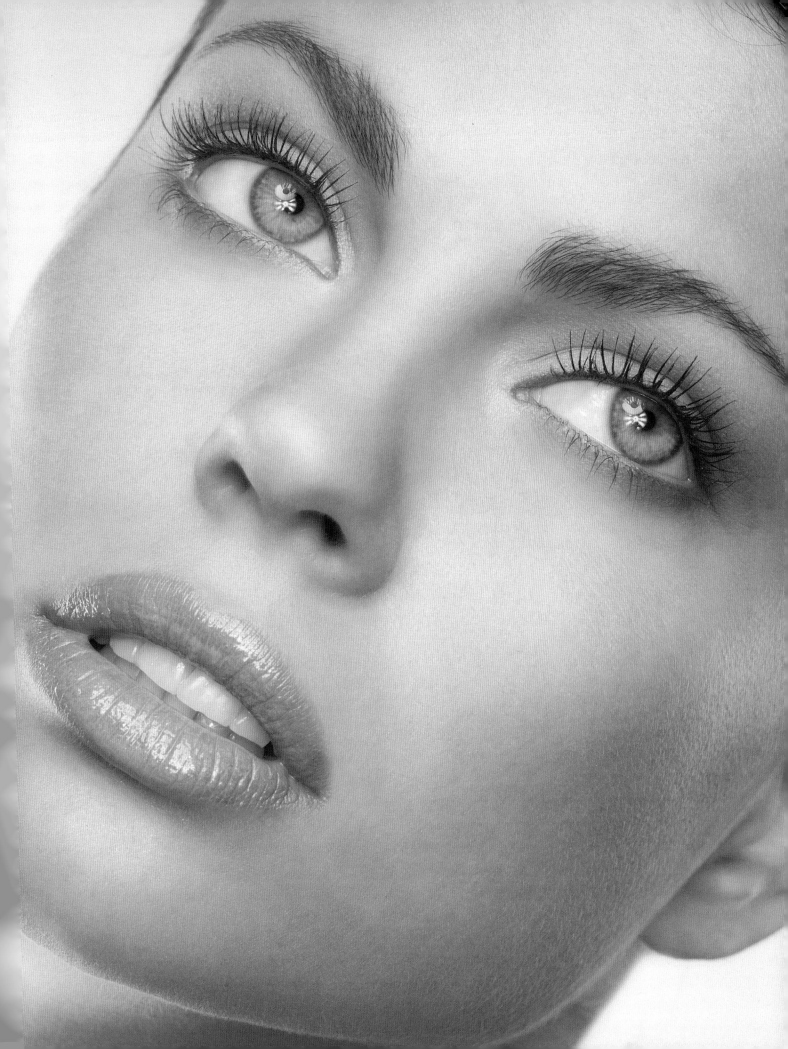

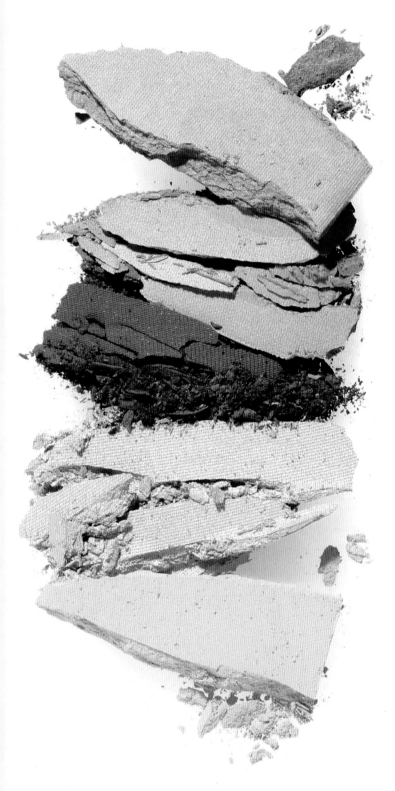

BLUSHING BRIDE

Want to be a rosy-cheeked, blushing bride? One of the most important things to think about, as I have already mentioned, is making sure your color lasts. Here's an easy way to layer your cheek color and make it last from the ceremony to the reception, photo after photo:

1. After applying your foundation, apply a crème blush to the apples of your cheeks and cheekbones.

2. Dust your face with loose or pressed powder.

3. Apply a powder blush (similar in color to the crème blush) to the apples of your cheeks and cheekbones.

Using this application method will give you a bit more intense color, and everything will last throughout the evening. Don't forget to bronze your cheeks: It will keep your skin looking warm and glowing throughout your entire wedding day. You will just have to bronze after you apply your blush with this application technique, because you need to apply your crème after your foundation and before you powder.

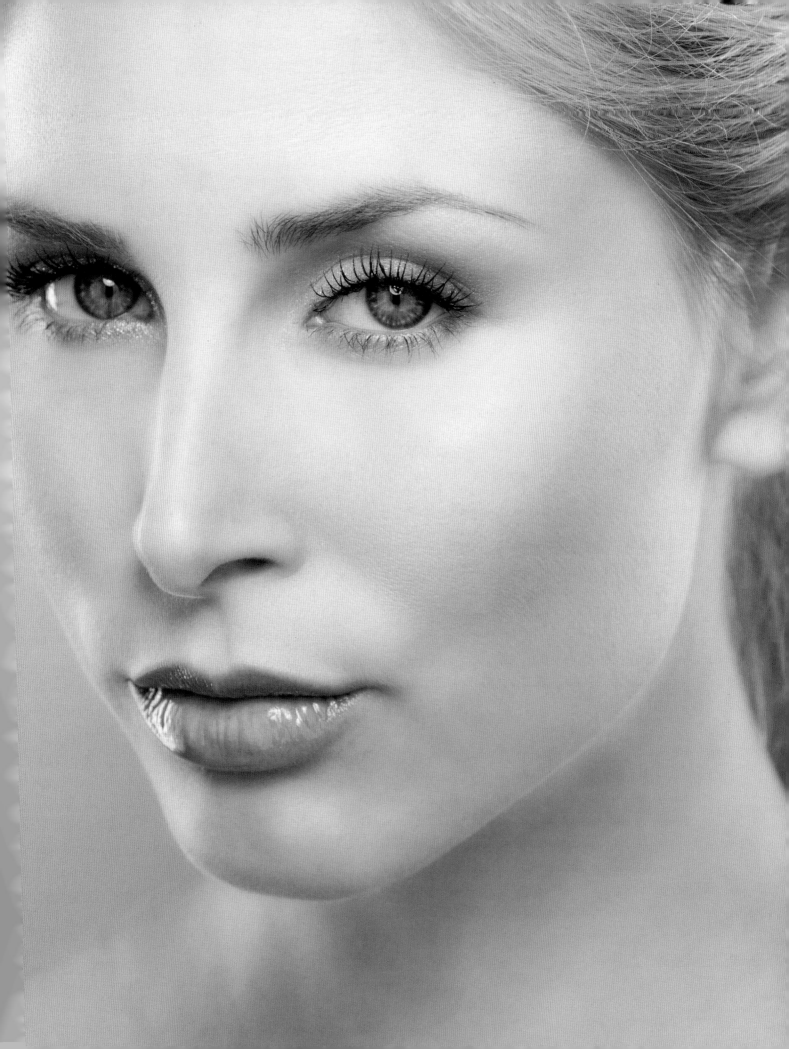

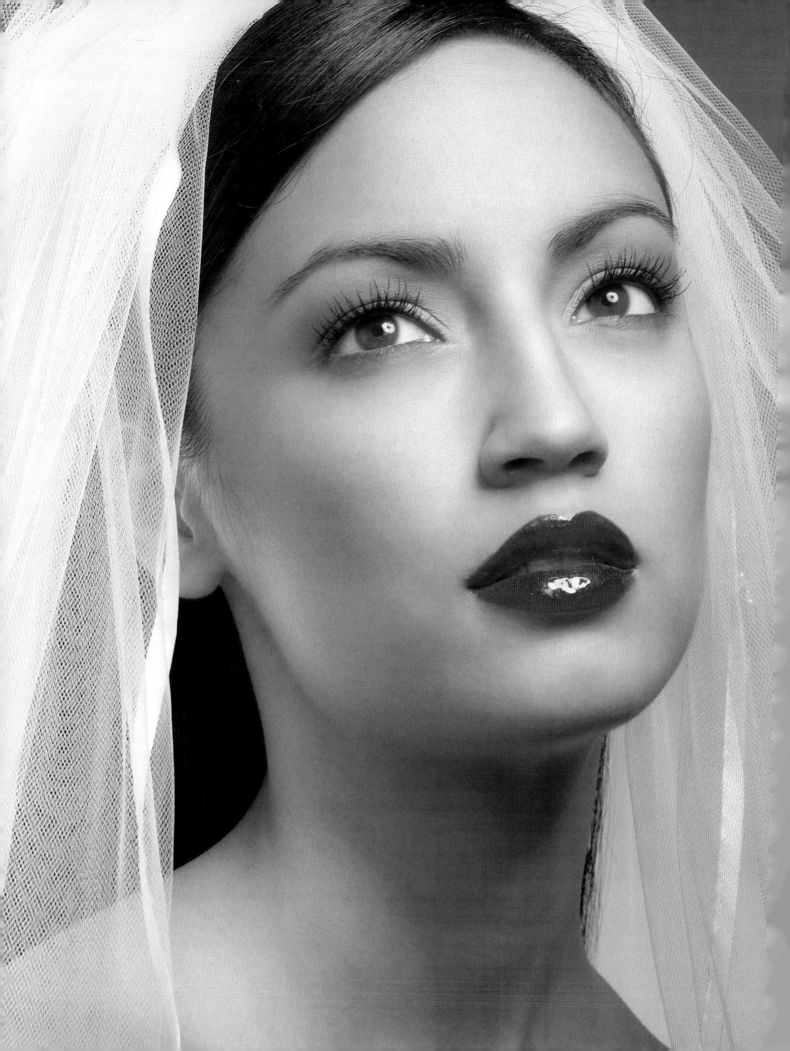

LIP COLOR THAT LASTS

Since it is your wedding day, you want to give your lip color "stay-ability" so your smile looks beautiful all day. You do *not* want to constantly be touching up your lips. This is a good time to buy two of your favorite lipstick and lip gloss —one set to keep in your makeup bag, and one to stash in the groom's pocket for quick lip fixes and instant pretty smiles.

There are many ways to get your lip color to last. I have tried them all, and I have found in the end that there is one that really works best:

1. Conceal the entire lip area, everything from the natural lip line to the actual lip. This will create a more perfect edge for photos by hiding any discoloration you might have just outside your lip line, as well as creating the perfect canvas on which to apply your lip color.

2. Line the outer edges of the lips with lip liner, then fill in the entire lip area with liner. This is the first line of defense in getting your lip color to last. Lip liner has a drier texture than lipstick, so it lasts longer.

3. Next, apply a soft, pretty lipstick that looks natural yet still defines the lips. Then, take a tissue and gently blot your lips. This will remove the moisture from this layer yet leave you with a deposit of pigment. Next, reapply your lipstick; this time, do not blot. Layering color like this will give you double the pigment deposit, thus increasing how long the color will last.

4. Finish with a dot of lip gloss in the center of the lips to attract light and highlight your smile for photographs. I have found that lips with a bit of shine to them photograph more beautifully because the shine gives them dimension in a photo.

5. If you only want to wear lip gloss, make sure to line your lips and fill in the entire lip with pencil before applying the gloss. This will help your lip gloss last longer.

One great quick tip: If you have a groom who is concerned about ending up wearing your lipstick after the kiss, lick your lips before you kiss him. This will prevent the color from transferring. If you are wearing lip gloss and do not want the color to transfer, have him lick his lips before he kisses you. Then none of the gloss will transfer, thus leaving his lips color-free.

I usually discourage brides from wearing a dark lip color on their wedding day. It doesn't photograph as well as softer, more natural shades. The only time I'm okay with a dark lip color is if the bride wears it daily and it is part of her everyday look. If you choose to wear a dark lip color, remember you must wear soft eye shades so the two features don't compete with each other.

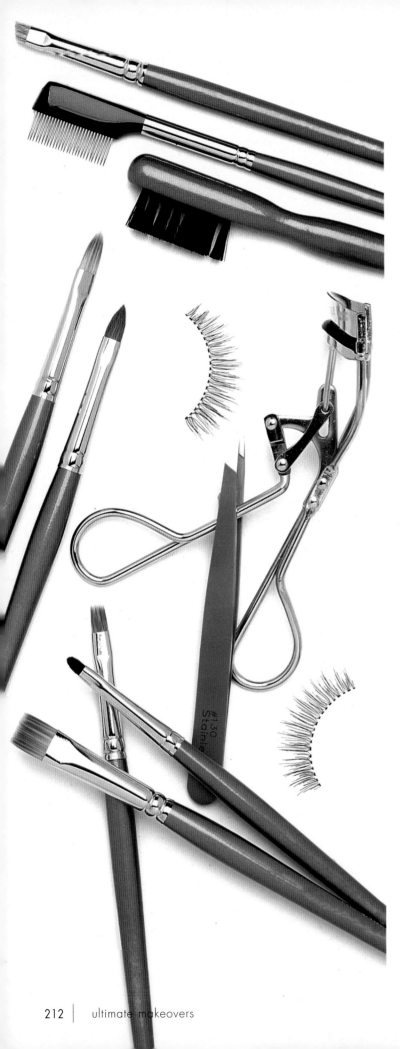

makeup must-haves

After you've decided on your look and favorite shades to wear, you'll want to pack your makeup bag with the beauty essentials on this list. The list contains everything you need to help you create a beautiful look and keep you looking radiant throughout your wedding day.

- moisturizer
- primer
- foundation
- concealer
- loose powder
- pressed powder
- bronzer
- brow color
- eyeliner
- eyelash curler
- mascara
- eye shadows
- false eyelashes (optional)
- blush
- lip pencil (2)
- lipstick (2)
- lip gloss (2)
- makeup brushes
- tweezers
- blotting papers
- sponges
- powder puff
- tissues

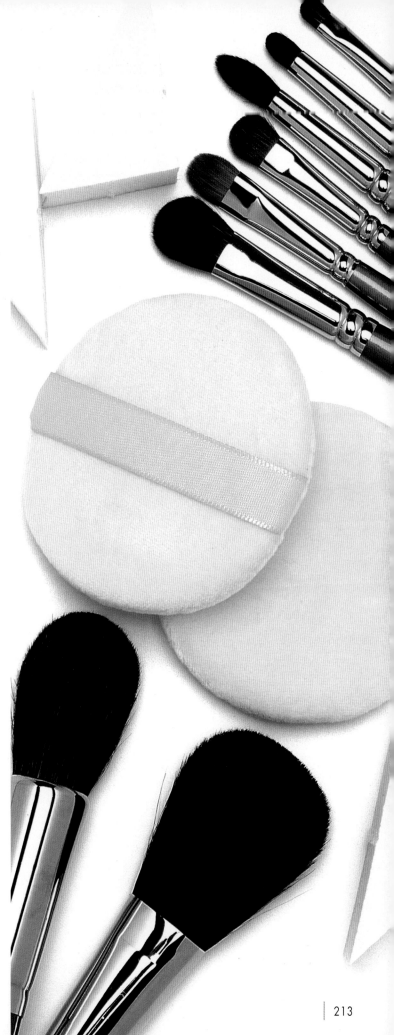

There are a few things on this list that I want to draw your attention to. Note that I've added the number "2" by a few of the products; you will need two of each of these products: one to put in your makeup bag for getting ready and one to use for touching up during the wedding.

Now I know most brides purchase a beautiful, expensive purse so you have a place to put your touchup makeup. But inevitably you gave the purse to Pam who gave to Tracey who gave it to Missy who gave it to Patty who can't remember where she put it, so when you need it, no one can find it.

I think the best place for those items is in the groom's jacket pocket. By the time you need them, you will be with him, and the darn purse is such a pain to keep up with anyway.

So the day before the wedding, give your groom your pressed powder, lip pencil, lipstick, lip gloss, and blotting papers to put in his pockets (he has at least three pockets). And if he is not willing to carry these small items for you, maybe you are marrying the wrong man!

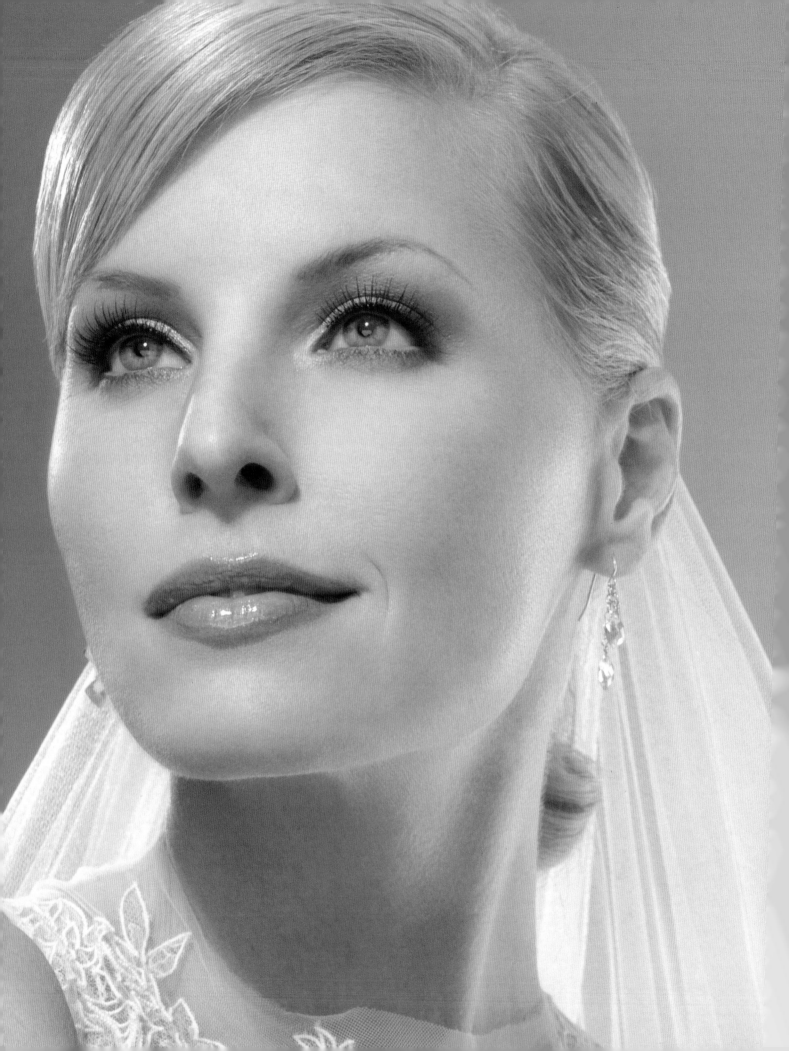

create your look

This day is all about you and how beautiful you are, so I want to help you create the perfect makeup look for you. In my experience, the one most important feature to spotlight on your wedding day is your eyes. As they say, they are the windows to your soul. Well-defined, beautiful eyes always photograph fabulously! Here are some amazing makeup looks you can use to create the perfect eye look for you. I have also given you blush and lipstick suggestions to help complete each look. As always, experiment with these looks, and have fun long before your wedding day! You can try one or all, and choose the one you like best.

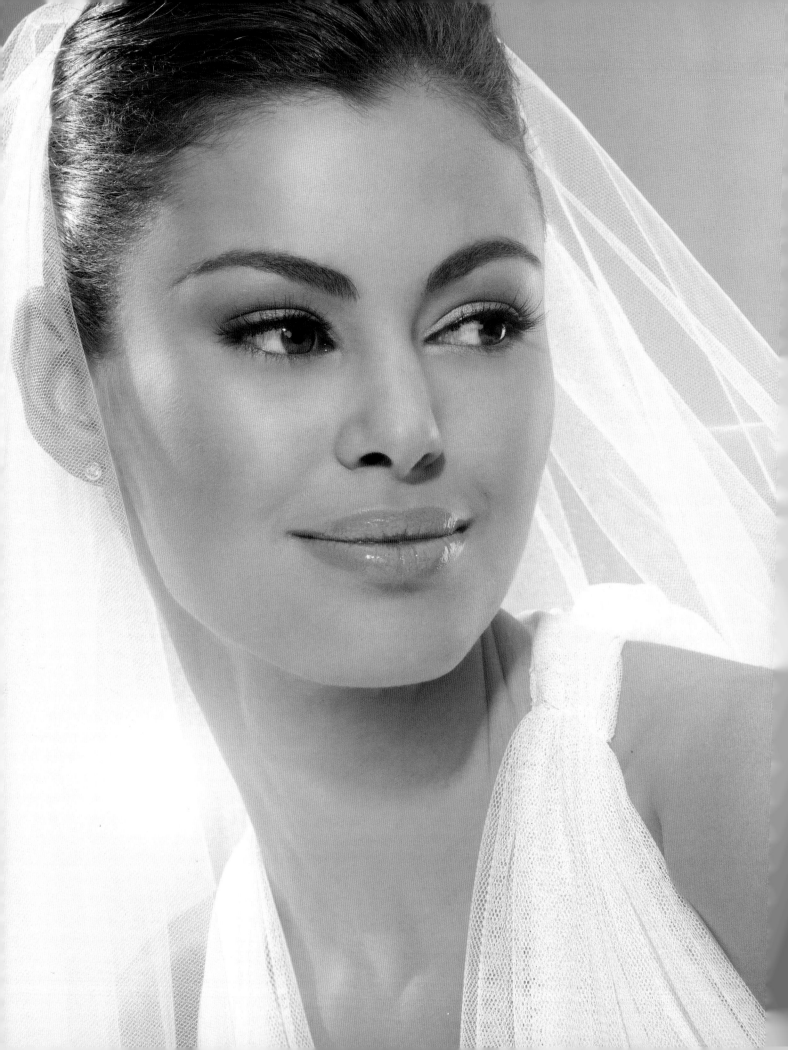

natural beauty

Eyeshadow is a great way to make the color of your eyes stand out and help define your eyes. If you simply want to bring out your natural beauty, this is a look that will be perfect for you. With this eyeshadow application, you can create everything from soft and natural to extremely dramatic, depending on your eyeshadow choices. To make sure you apply your shadows properly, follow the steps below for a simple application that will shape your eyelids and make you feel absolutely beautiful.

It takes three shades of eyeshadow to shape the eye: a highlight, midtone, and contour shade. Depending on the effect you want to achieve, your eyeshadow choices will make a big difference in the way you look. If you want to look soft and natural, choose soft colors; if you want to look more dramatic, choose a contour shade that is deeper and richer in color.

APPLICATION:

1. Highlight shade: Apply to browbone, the lid, and inside corner of lower lashline.

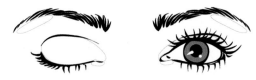

2. Midtone shade: Starting from the outside corner of the eyelid (because the first place you lay your brush gets the most color) gently move your brush across the crease into the inside corner of the eyelid. Also brush along the lower lashline, once again starting from the outside corner and brushing toward the inside, so that the most intense color is at the outside, fading as you move to the inside corner. This will help you create subtle definition.

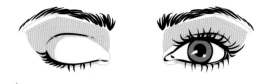

3. Contour shade: Apply across your upper lashline from the outside corner inward. Then bring the color up into the outer portion of the crease, and blend it inward about one third of the way, layering it on top of your midtone shade. Sweep color underneath the lower lashline for a soft, blended look.

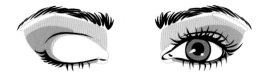

With this look, you have a multitude of blush and lip color options, depending on the intensity of eyeshadow you choose. For instance, if you choose a dark eyeshadow contour color, make sure you choose soft and subtle lip and blush colors. If you choose really soft and natural eyeshadow colors, you could choose a bit more intense lip and blush colors.

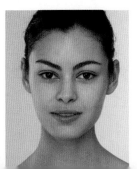

audrey hepburn eye

For a very sophisticated bride, this application technique will give you a simply beautiful look. This look is a modern take on the classic Audrey Hepburn look from *Breakfast at Tiffany's*. In the classic version of this look, there is no color along the bottom lashline. However, in our modern version, we are using your midtone eyeshadow shade to help create definition. This look is always beautiful and sophisticated.

APPLICATION:

1. Highlight shade: Apply to the browbone and the lid. Highlight the inside corner underneath the lower lashline (wrap the color around the inside corner of the eye) for added drama.

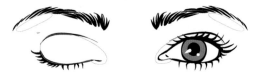

2. Midtone shade: Starting in the crease, apply your midtone color from the outer to the inner corner of the eye. Sweep the same color underneath the lower lashline for definition.

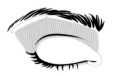 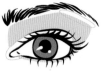

3. Eyeliner: Start by taking an eyeliner pencil and lining the upper eyelid first to start your pattern (perfect line). Start at the inside corner of the eye, and kick the liner upward at the outer corner. Make sure the line increases from thin to thick as you go toward the outer corner. Next, using a black shadow and an eyeliner brush, go over your pencil and fine-tune it, making it the perfect shape. Then follow the line with liquid eyeliner. Since you have first created the perfect pattern and then applied your liquid liner on top, if it is not perfect, no one will know, because you created the perfect shape first with your pencil and powder.

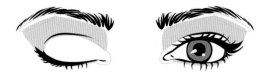

4. To really finish this look, apply false eyelashes. See page 206 for easy application steps.

When choosing a blush to go with this style of eye makeup, just remember that this is a classic look, so do not choose anything too strong or it could overpower your eyes. Unlike your blush, your lip choice could be a bit stronger with this eye look. Since it is soft and subtle, a little more intense lip color could look very sophisticated.

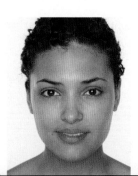

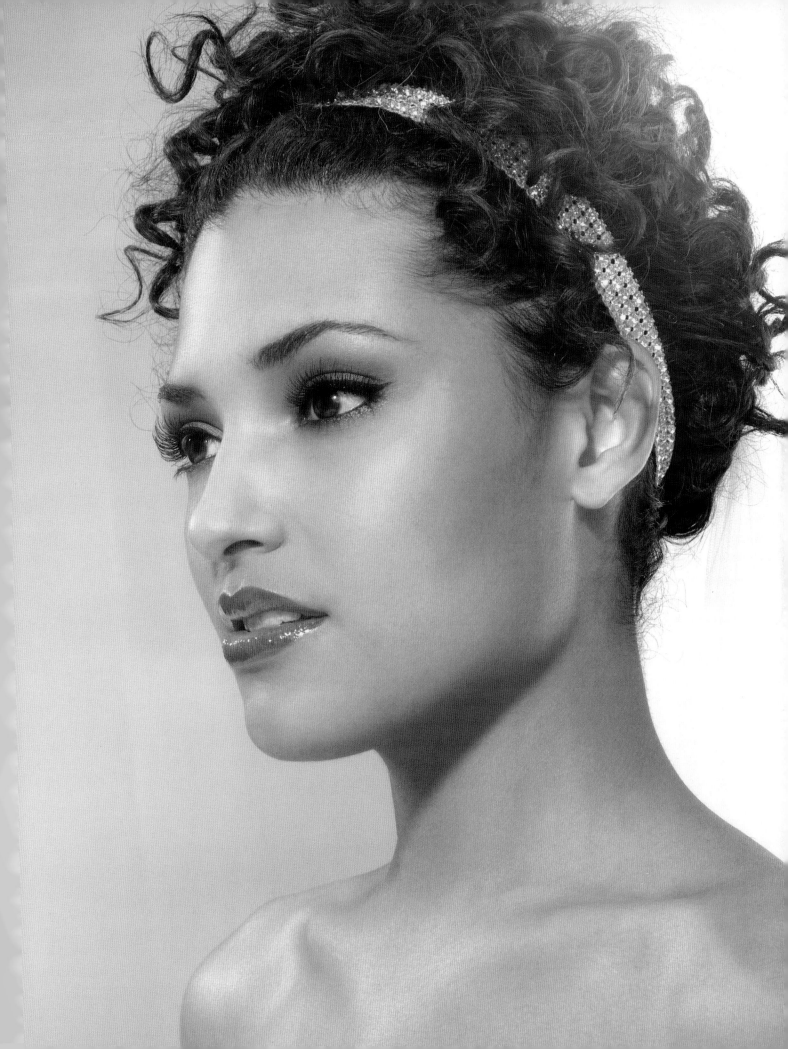

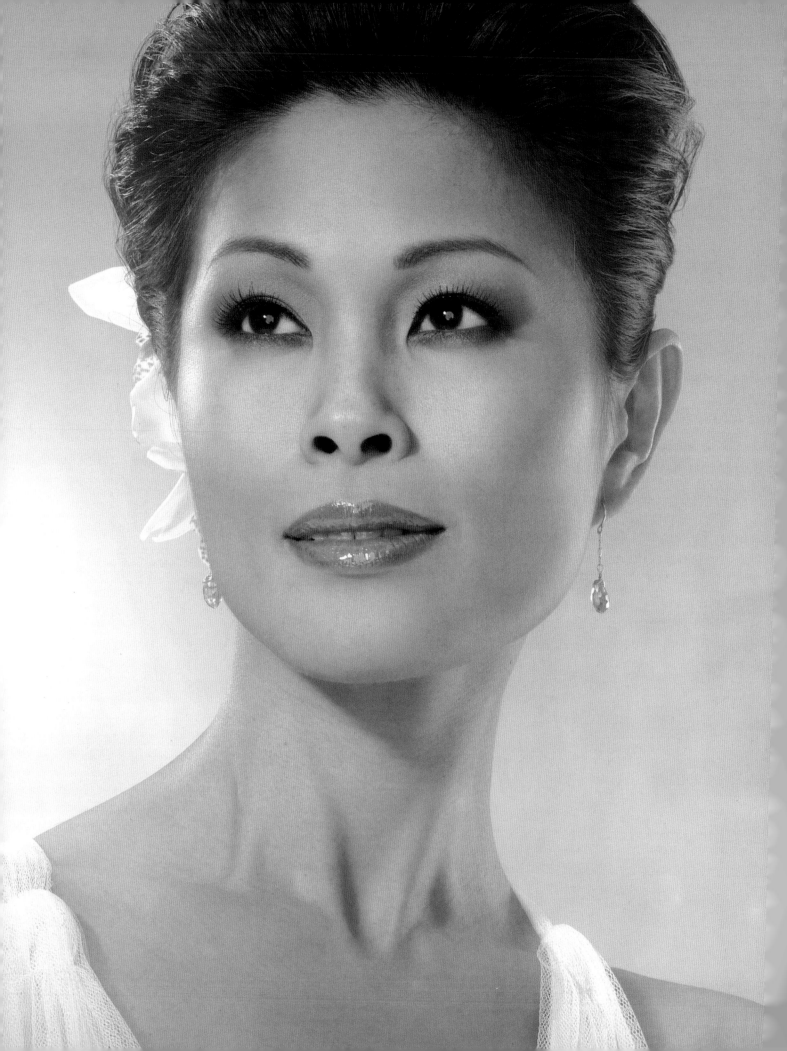

smoky eye

This look is perfect for the bride who wants a more dramatic look on her day. With this application technique, you will be able to create a sexy, smoky eye. Even though this is definitely a dramatic look, you control just how dramatic it is by choosing how dark your eyeshadow shades will be. You can use lighter shades and create a subtle effect, or choose darker shades for maximum drama. Whatever your eyeshadow color choice is, this application technique will define your eyes and make you look gorgeous in photographs.

APPLICATION:

1. Highlight shade: Apply to browbone only.

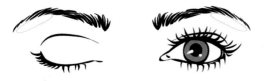

2. Midtone shade: Start at the base of your upper lashline, and bring the color up and over your entire lid—all the way up to your browbone. Also brush it along the lower lashline. This will help to create definition.

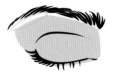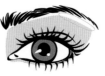

3. Contour shade: Again, start at the base of your lashline, and layer the color over your midtone all the way across your lid and up into the crease. Now sweep the contour color underneath the lower lashline as well. You'll create a light-to-dark effect with the three eyeshadows, with the darkest shade applied closest to the lashline and fading as you go toward the brow.

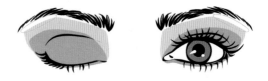

4. With this look, make sure you line your entire eye all along the top and bottom lashline.

With the smoky eye look, your eyes are the absolute focus. Soft, subtly glowing cheeks would look best. You can use color—just make sure it is a soft, sheer color so that it is not too intense for the eyes. If you choose deep, rich eyeshadow colors, make sure you wear a very soft, subtle lip color. You never want both your eyes and lips to be dark! Your lips should be as subtle as possible; close to nude would be best. It would look fantastic if you chose just to wear a really soft, beautiful lip gloss with this look. A soft gloss color would not be too strong and fight with your eyes for attentiona.

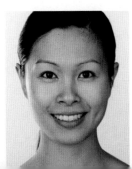

sparkling eye

Put a twinkle in your eye and give yourself a fresh glowing look. Nothing is more beautiful than a look with a bit of sparkle and shine to the eye. The key to this look is to create the shine or sparkle on only the eye. You want to make sure the rest of your face has very little shine to it. Your skin should be matte, your blush should have no shimmer to it, and your lips should not be too glossy. The only shade that should have shimmer to it is your highlight shadow.

APPLICATION:

1. Highlight shade: Apply a sparkly highlight shade to your browbone and lid. Make sure to highlight the "V" on the inside corner of the eye (wrap the color around the inside corner). This will really accentuate the shimmer and sparkle.

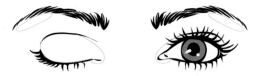

2. Midtone shade: Starting from the outside corner of the crease, sweep the color across to the inside corner of your eye. Also brush it along the lower lashline, once again starting from the outside corner and brushing toward the inside, so that the most intense color is at the outside, fading as you move to the inside corner. This will help you create subtle definition. Make sure this shade is matte.

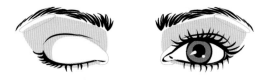

3. Contour shade: Sweep the color along the upper lashline and into the crease, layering it on top of your midtone shade. Apply underneath the eye all along the lower lashline. Make sure this shade is also matte.

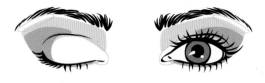

When making blush and lip choices, you want to make sure you don't overpower the sparkly eye that you have just created. Remember: no shimmer to your blush! Make sure you choose a soft, subtle shade that will give your cheeks a glow. You can wear a lip gloss if you like, but make sure that it will not overpower your eyes.

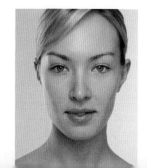

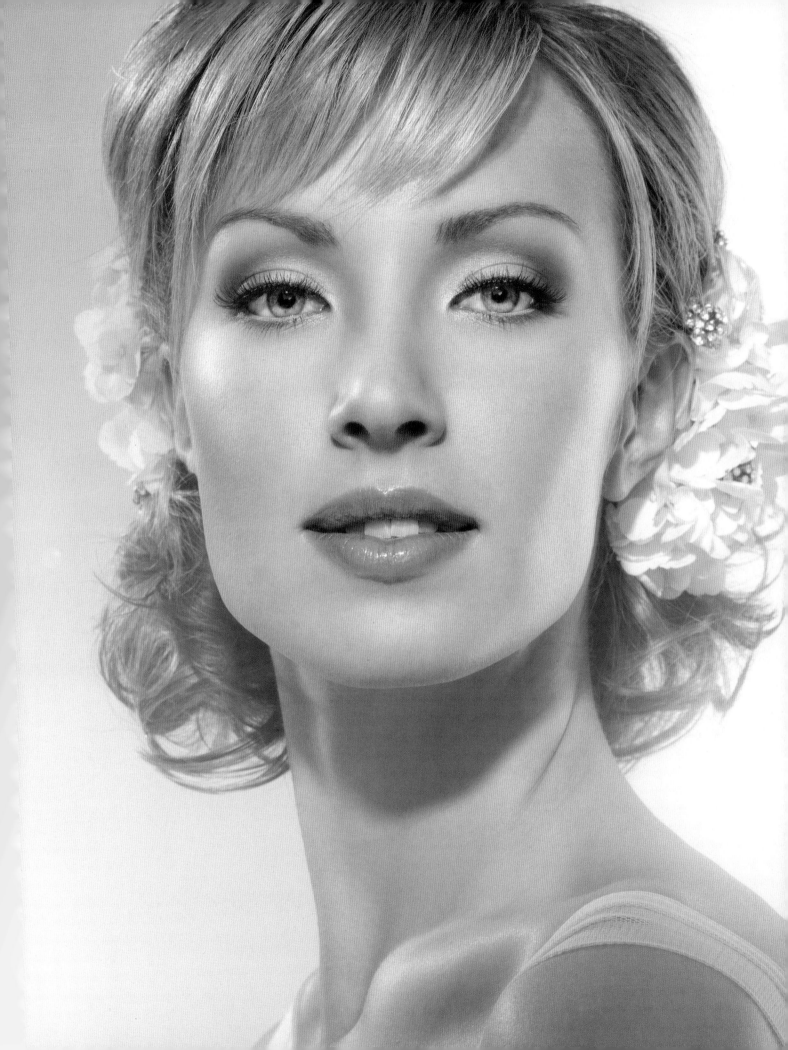

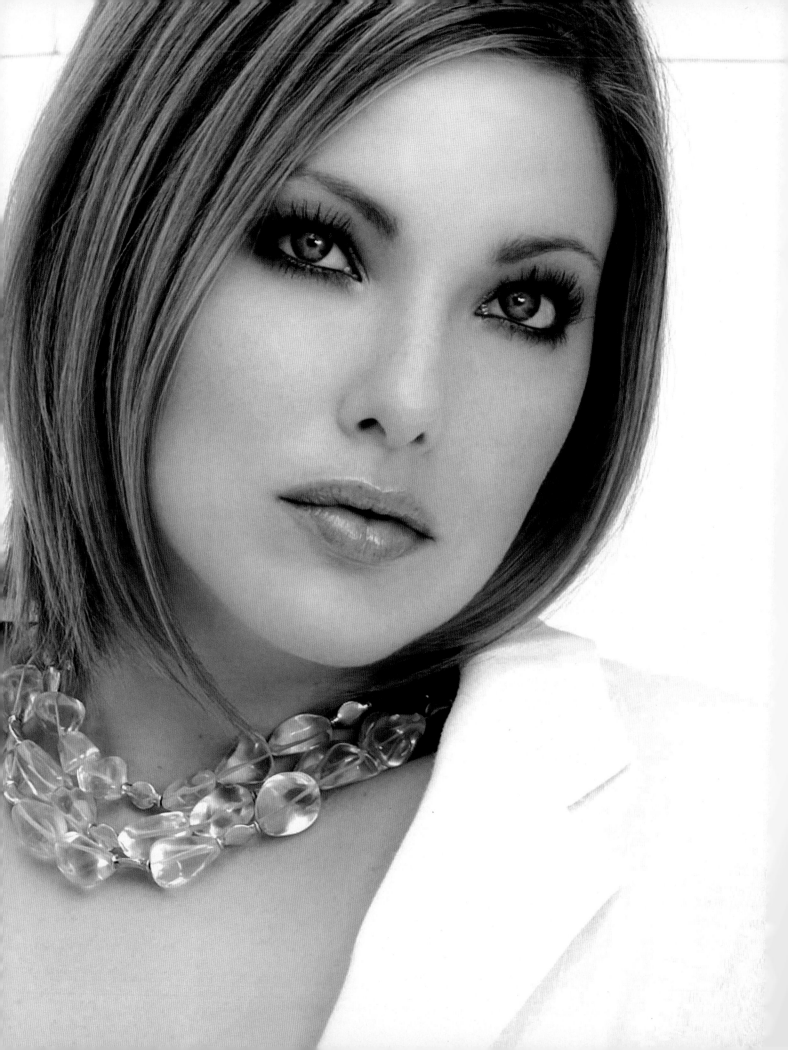

matte	nude	highlight		matte	ginger	midtone	
matte	sand	highlight		matte	mahogany	midtone	
shimmer	flesh	highlight		shimmer	pinkish brown	contour	
shimmer	beige	highlight		shimmer	purple	contour	
shimmer	gold	highlight		shimmer	chocolate	contour	
shimmer	coral	highlight		shimmer	golden brown	contour	
matte	taupe	midtone		shimmer	burgundy	contour	
matte	rose	midtone		matte	mahogany	contour	
matte	dark taupe	midtone		matte	dark brown	contour	
matte	caramel	midtone		matte	charcoal	contour	

I have put together a comprehensive chart of eyeshadow colors that I have used to create all the looks in part four. I've given you a palette with a wide array of colors, so every woman can find a look that she will love.

The names are generic, so you can compare with any cosmetic line and find these shades. Simply by using the chart on this page, you can see what specific eyeshadow shades I used to create all the bridal looks in chapter 18.

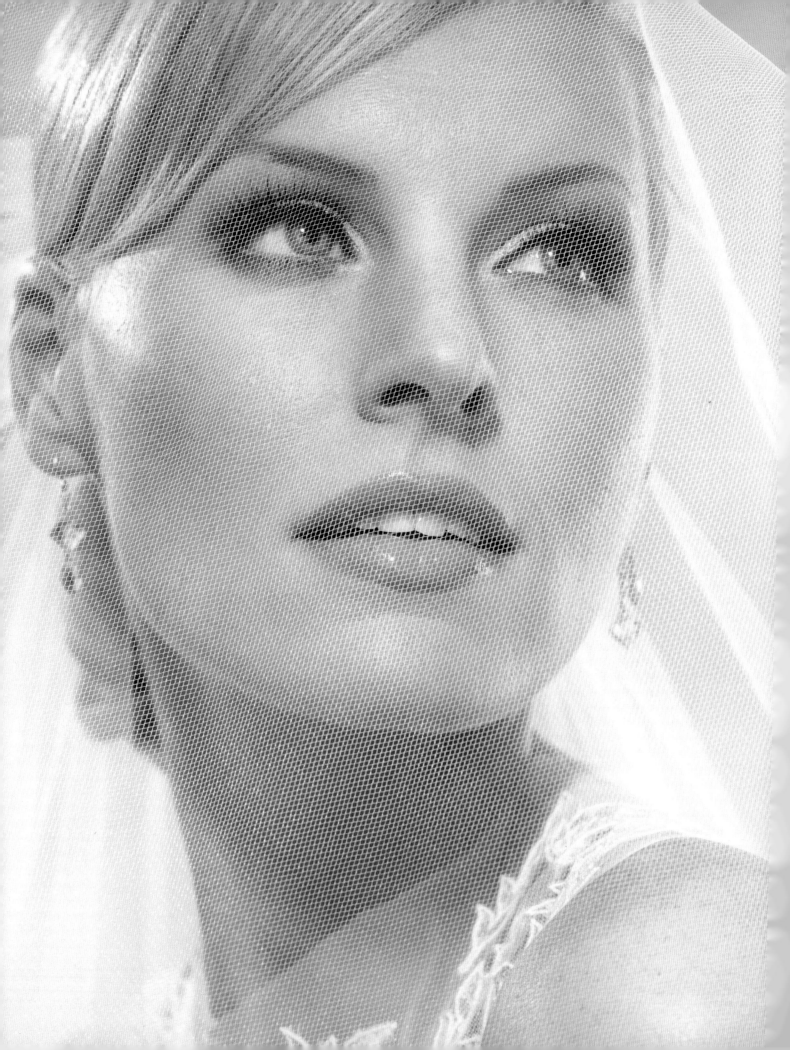

pictureperfect

In my opinion, the most important thing to think about when preparing for your wedding is how you will photograph. Many, many years from now, when the wedding dress no longer fits, the only tangible thing you will have to really remember your special day are the photographs. So when considering your makeup look for your wedding photos or your bridal portrait, remember that it's all about making your best features stand out in the photo. You want to define your features better—not cover everything up with heavier makeup.

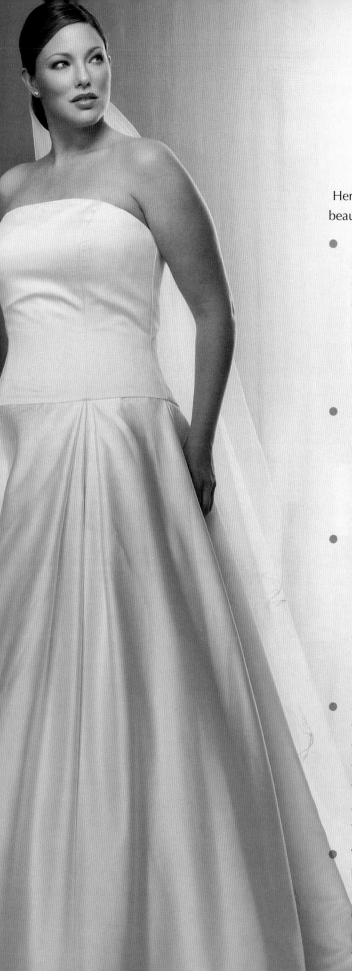

Here are a few tips that can help you create beautiful wedding photos and bridal portraits.

● If you're posing for a bridal portrait in a studio, you can wear more makeup than you could if you were taking your photographs outside, because you don't have the different lighting factors to consider. If you are posing outside, you'll want to review the tips in chapter 14 on natural lighting and how it can affect your look at different times of day.

● Make sure to warm up your skin and give it dimension by sculpting and bronzing your face. To review tips on how to sculpt the face, turn to page 83. To review how to use bronzing powder for that perfect glow, turn to page 140.

● If you want to wear foundation and powder with a bit of sheen to it, you may do so if your portrait is taken in a studio (but remember that matte skin always photographs more flawlessly). But stick with a matte look for your wedding day or if your portrait is being taken outside (due to the different lighting situations).

● Blush adds life to the face. You may choose to wear a shade that's a bit more colorful for your portrait than you choose to wear on your wedding day. Even if you do not normally wear blush every day, you will want to wear at least a little color for photographs to give your face a bit of life.

● Warmer cheek colors photograph more beautifully than cool colors, because they make the skin look fresh and glowing. But don't forget that applying a little bronzing powder first will give you a fresh glow that will make you look unforgettable.

- You can wear matte or shimmer eyeshadows for your portrait and your wedding day but never frosted shadows. They always look too shiny and artificial in photographs. Remember, this picture is forever!

- Make sure at least one of your eyeshadows has a matte finish. Generally, you never want to use three shades of shadow with a shimmer because they will make the lid look too shiny. It is okay, however, to use three matte shades. For me, the one shade I almost always choose to be matte is my midtone, because it is supposed to look the most natural.

- When choosing eyeshadows for photography, shades with warm undertones (including brown) enhance every eye color and will photograph beautifully.

- Don't choose shades that are too bold. This is not the time for bright fuchsia lipstick or charcoal eyeshadow. Instead, you should choose lip shades that are just a few shades darker than your natural lip tone. Select eyeshadow shades that are deep enough to create definition and enhance your eye color, but not dark enough to demand all the attention. Your goal is to define your features with enough color to see the definition in the photographs, but not so much that you overwhelm and distort your features.

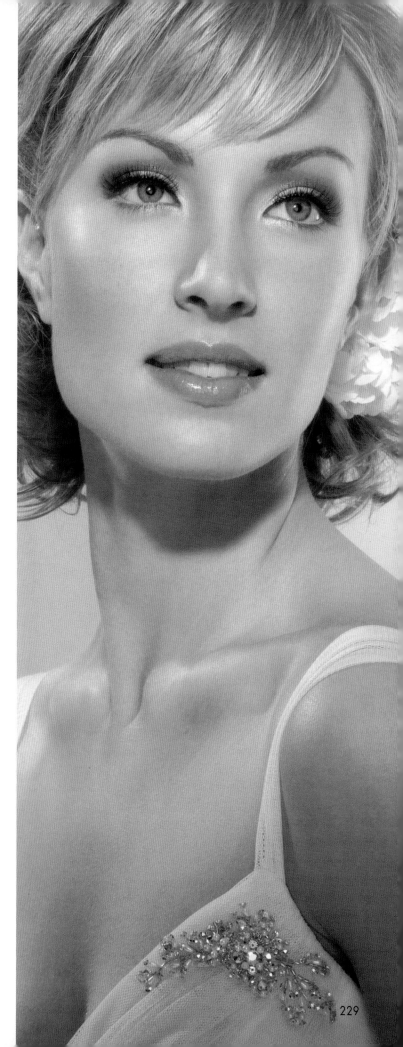

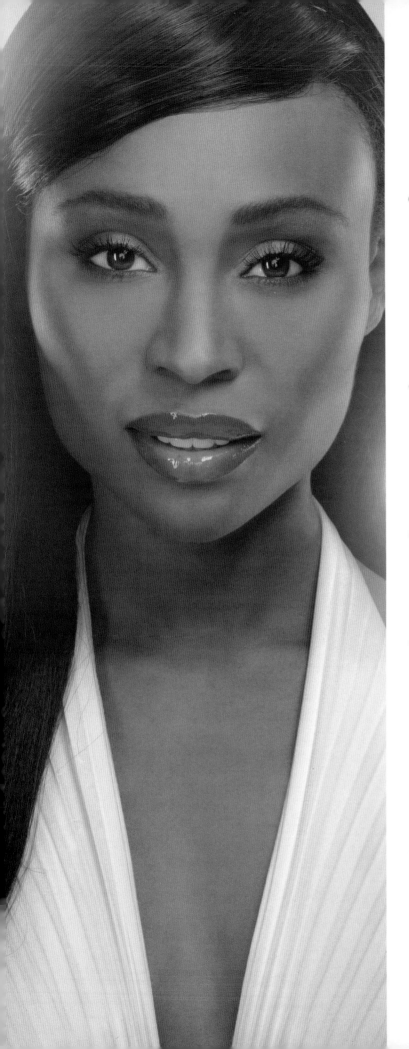

- Nothing will bring out your eyes better in a photograph than defining really well at the lashline. There are two ways to achieve this. First, you could layer your mascara to help thicken and lengthen your lashes. Turn to page 135 to learn how. The second technique—and my favorite for the absolute best definition—is to apply false eyelashes. Turn to page 206 for foolproof application tips.

- Make sure your lips are well defined for your portrait. Erasing your natural lip line with foundation or concealer before you apply your color will give you a fresh, perfect canvas, so that when you apply your lip liner it will give your lips perfect definition in photographs.

- Brows should be well groomed and defined with brow color. Even if you do not normally wear eyebrow color, in a photograph, the light could possibly wash your brows out, so a little color for definition might be necessary.

- I know I have already mentioned it, but I want to end by reminding you again that powder is your friend when you're being photographed. Matte skin always photographs more flawlessly than shiny skin!

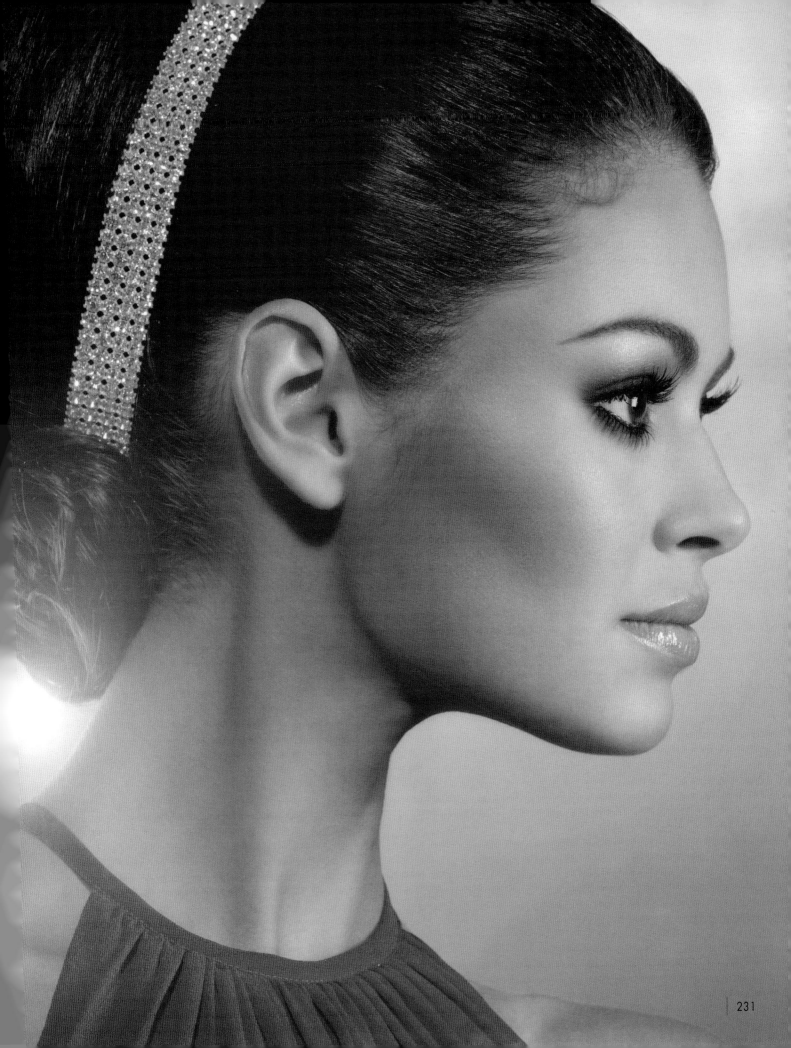

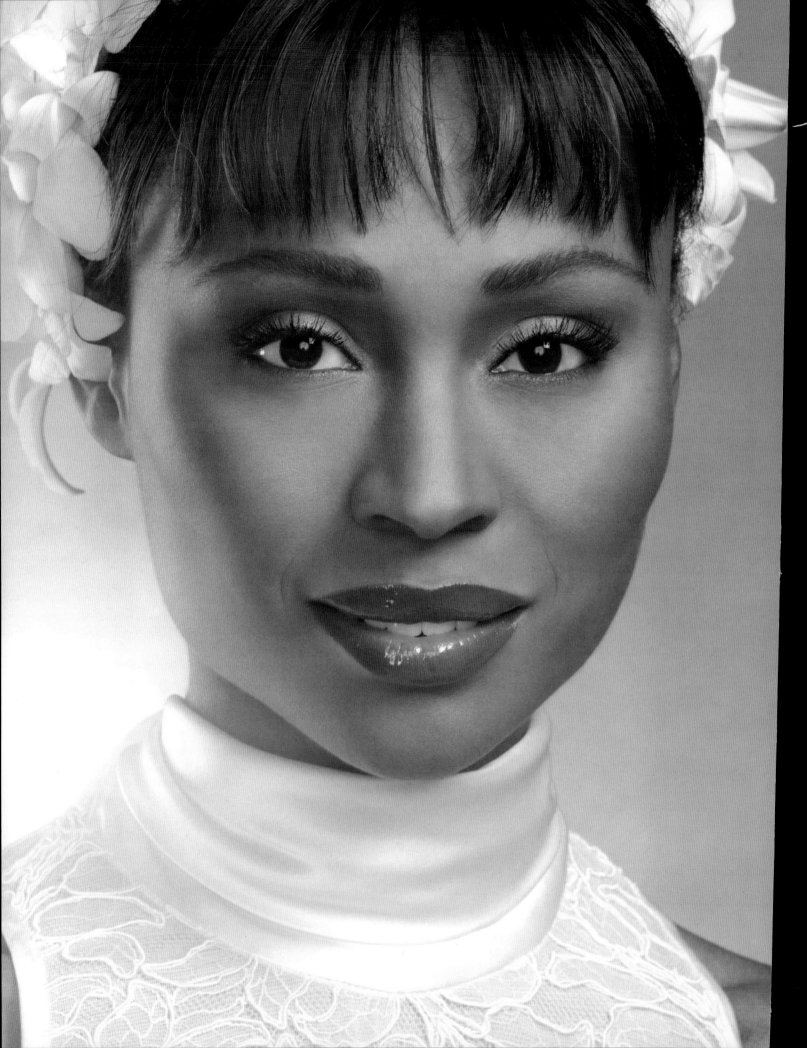

bridalinspiration

In this chapter, I have gathered together some before and after photographs to show what makeup looks really work to make a beautiful bride. I have listed the eyeshadow applications I have used for each look as well as the time or times of day these looks will photograph most beautifully. I have also listed the blush and lipstick shades used. With all this information, you will surely be able to create the perfect look for you! Remember to try many different looks before your wedding, since you never know what you might discover.

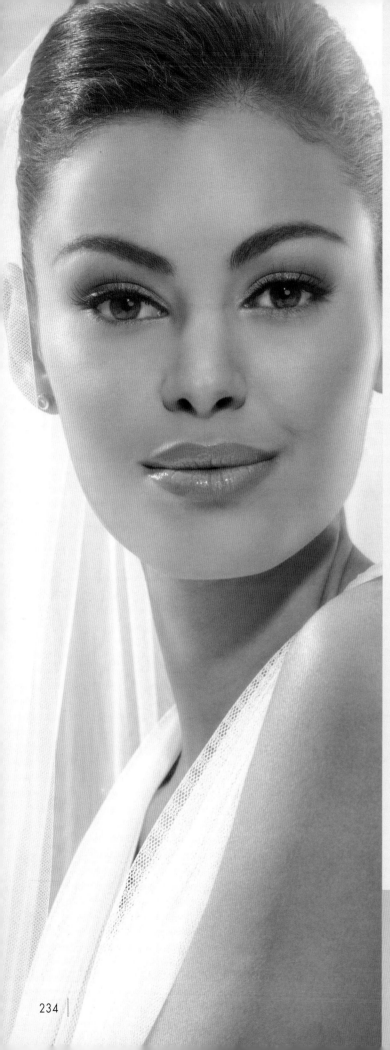

nonna

WEDDING TIME:	morning/midday/ late afternoon/evening
EYESHADOW APPLICATION:	natural beauty (page 217)
EYESHADOW:	highlight: shimmer beige midtone: matte taupe contour: shimmer pinkish brown
EYELINER:	taupe
BLUSH:	rich honey
LIP LINER:	flesh
LIPSTICK:	pinkish nude
LIP GLOSS:	creamy nude
TIPS:	This look works perfectly for any time of day, because it is so subtle yet it defines every feature. Notice how I really achieved a lot of definition on the eyes with thick, dark long lashes. Choosing subtle lip and blush colors gives the entire look a beautiful natural appeal.

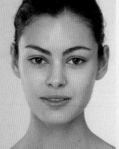

eleanor

WEDDING TIME:	late afternoon/evening
EYESHADOW APPLICATION:	smoky eye (page 221)
EYESHADOW:	highlight: shimmer gold midtone: matte caramel contour: shimmer burgundy
EYELINER:	rich brown
BLUSH:	rich honey
LIP LINER:	warm caramel
LIPSTICK:	soft peach
LIP GLOSS:	shimmer coral
TIPS:	Normally I would only let a bride wear a smoky eye during an evening wedding, but because I chose softer eyeshadow shades and still used a smoky eye application, she could also wear this look for a late afternoon wedding. Don't forget that a subtle lip shade will still be the best choice.

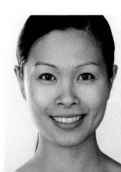

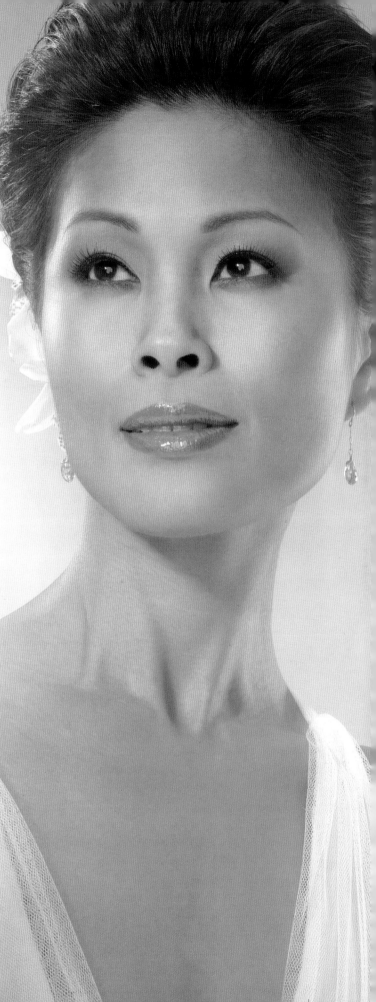

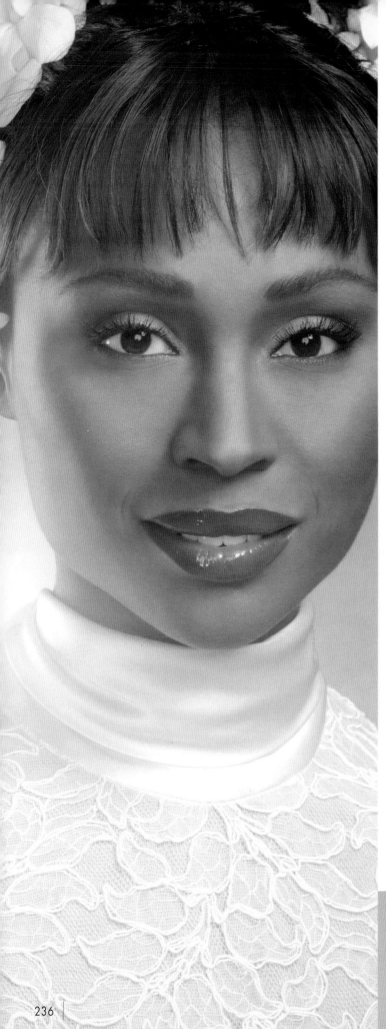

cynthia

WEDDING TIME:	morning/midday/ late afternoon/evening
EYESHADOW APPLICATION:	natural beauty (page 217)
EYESHADOW:	highlight: shimmer coral midtone: matte ginger contour: shimmer chocolate
EYELINER:	rich brown
BLUSH:	rich terracotta
LIP LINER:	warm caramel
LIPSTICK:	golden nude
LIP GLOSS:	shimmer bronze
TIPS:	Because this look is so natural yet defines every feature, it is perfect for any time of day. What makes it so versatile is the fact that my shade choices are subtle and natural but still add all the definition a bride needs, even for an evening wedding.

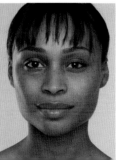

marisol

WEDDING TIME:	late afternoon/evening
EYESHADOW APPLICATION:	natural beauty (page 217)
EYESHADOW:	highlight: shimmer flesh midtone: matte taupe contour: matte dark taupe
EYELINER:	taupe
BLUSH:	rich honey
LIP LINER:	burgundy
LIPSTICK:	rich berry
LIP GLOSS:	shimmer berry
TIPS:	I would normally never do a dark lip for a wedding. But since it is a part of Marisol's everyday look, it is appropriate for her. I still kept in mind the time of day of the wedding, though. If it had been a morning or midday wedding, it would have been a "no go" on the dark lip!

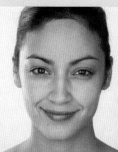

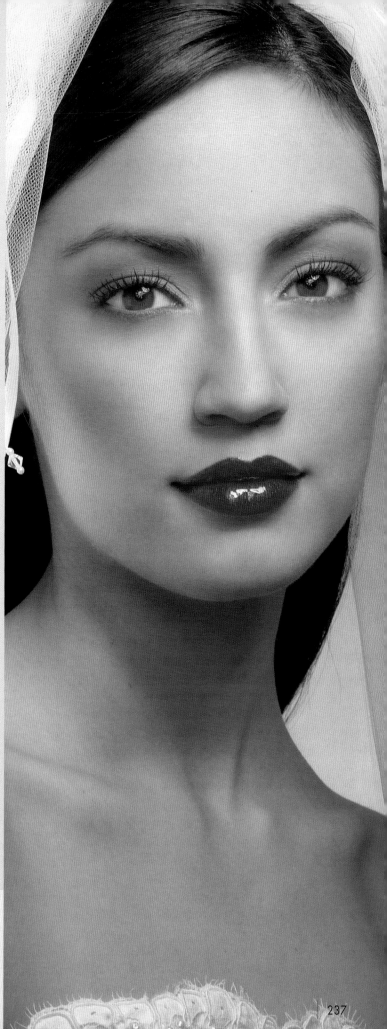

237

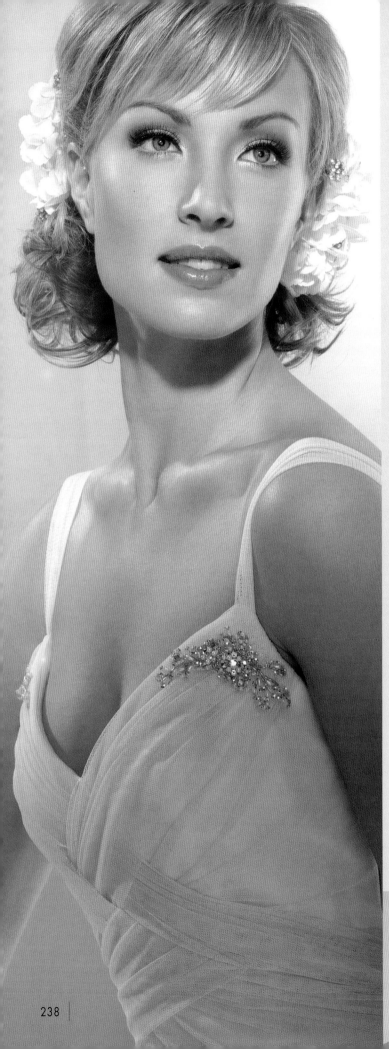

kate

WEDDING TIME:	midday/late afternoon/evening
EYESHADOW APPLICATION:	sparkling eye (page 222)
EYESHADOW:	highlight: matte nude/ shimmer flesh midtone: matte taupe contour: matte dark brown
EYELINER:	rich brown
BLUSH:	warm pink
LIP LINER:	flesh
LIPSTICK:	warm pink
LIP GLOSS:	creamy nude
TIPS:	To make the shimmer highlight eyeshadow shade show the most, I first layered a matte nude color on the lid (to create a base), then applied the shimmer highlight eyeshadow shade on top to make it stand out even more. Notice that I still concentrated on creating a really strong defining line at the lashline for the most intense definition.

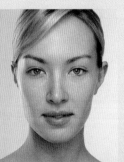

carol

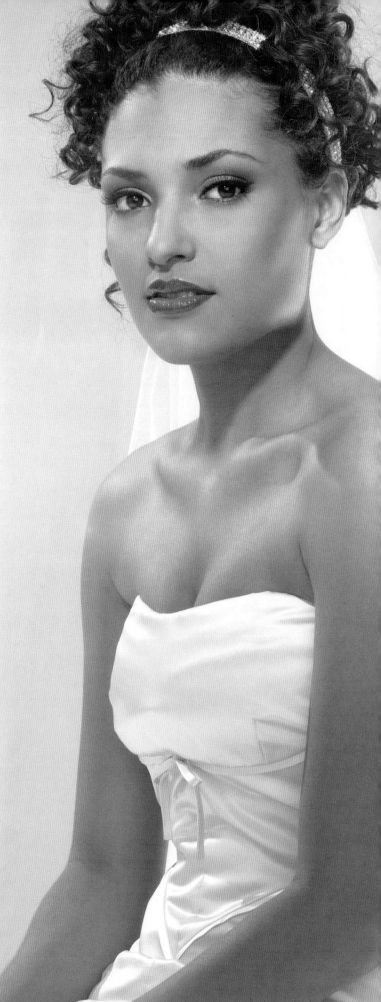

WEDGING TIME:	morning/midday/ late afternoon/evening
EYESHADOW APPLICATION:	audrey hepburn eye (page 218)
EYESHADOW:	highlight: shimmer gold midtone: shimmer pinkish brown
EYELINER:	charcoal
BLUSH:	rich terracotta
LIP LINER:	warm caramel
LIPSTICK:	golden nude
LIP GLOSS:	shimmer berry
TIPS:	Carol's look works at any time of day because it is a classic. But I have taken that classic look and given it a modern twist. You can never go wrong with simply being beautiful!

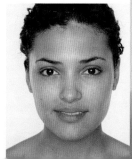

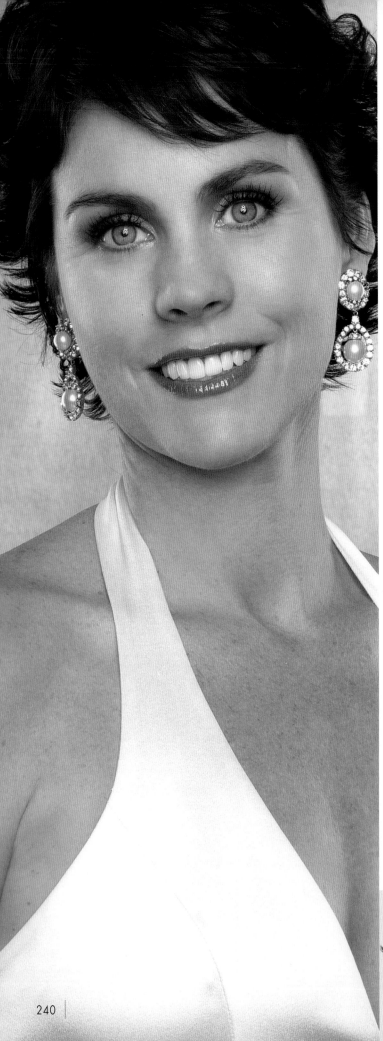

jamie

WEDDING TIME:	morning/midday/ late afternoon/evening
EYESHADOW APPLICATION:	natural beauty (page 217)
EYESHADOW:	highlight: shimmer beige midtone: matte taupe contour: shimmer golden brown
EYELINER:	bronze
BLUSH:	soft apricot
LIP LINER:	warm caramel
LIPSTICK:	warm pink
LIP GLOSS:	shimmer warm pink
TIPS:	Jamie's look is simple and natural, which is one reason it works at any time. I put the most intense eyeshadow colors at the base of the lashes. This will give Jamie's eyes the definition that I am looking for, but still keep her looking soft and natural.

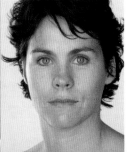

gayle

WEDDING TIME:	late afternoon/evening
EYESHADOW APPLICATION:	sparkling eye (page 222)
EYESHADOW:	highlight: shimmer beige midtone: matte caramel contour: matte dark brown
EYELINER:	rich brown
BLUSH:	rich honey
LIP LINER:	warm caramel
LIPSTICK:	soft peach
LIP GLOSS:	shimmer coral
TIPS:	To make the shimmer highlight eyeshadow shade show the most, I first layered a matte nude color on the lid (to create a base), then applied the shimmer highlight eyeshadow shade on top to make it stand out even more. Normally, a sparkling eyeshadow application will work at any time of day, but because I chose eyeshadow shades that are a bit deeper, Gayle's look would be best for late afternoon or evening.

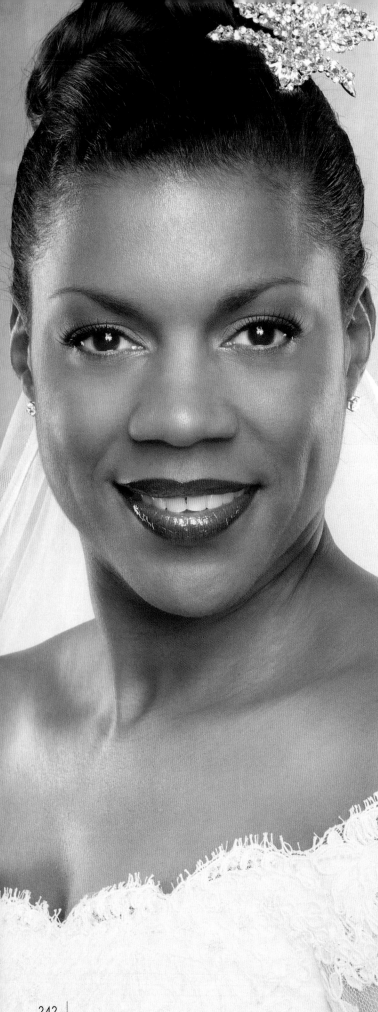

maxine

WEDDING TIME:	midday/late afternoon/evening
EYESHADOW APPLICATION:	natural beauty (page 217)
EYESHADOW:	highlight: shimmer gold midtone: matte mahogany contour: shimmer burgundy
EYELINER:	rich brown
BLUSH:	rich terracotta
LIP LINER:	burgundy
LIPSTICK:	rich berry
LIP GLOSS:	shimmer berry
TIPS:	For Maxine's look, I chose to make her lips the attention-getter, rather than her eyes. That is why I chose a bit darker and richer lip color and chose slightly softer eyeshadow colors.

missy

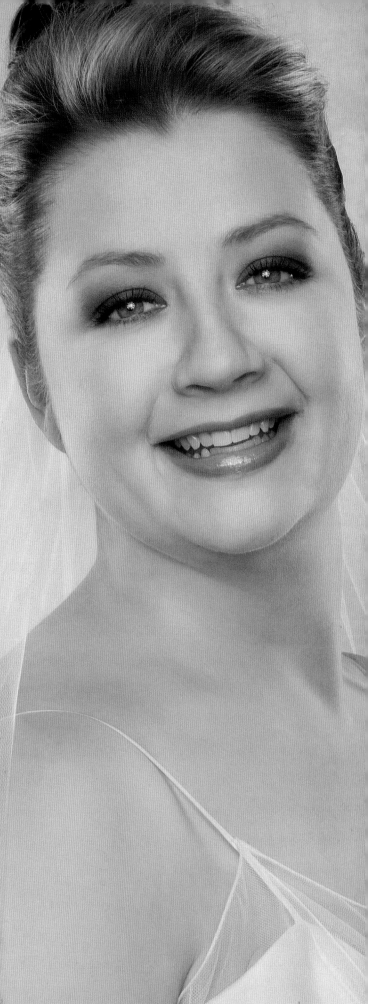

WEDDING TIME:	late afternoon/evening
EYESHADOW APPLICATION:	smoky eye (page 221)
EYESHADOW:	highlight: shimmer flesh midtone: matte taupe contour: matte mahogany
EYELINER:	rich brown
BLUSH:	soft peach
LIP LINER:	warm caramel
LIPSTICK:	soft peach
LIP GLOSS:	shimmer coral
TIPS:	Normally, I would only let a bride wear a smoky eye during an evening wedding, but because I chose softer eyeshadow shades and still used a smoky eye application, Missy could also wear this look for a late afternoon wedding. But don't forget that, even though we have used soft eyeshadow shades, we must still keep the lip soft so as not to overpower the bride!

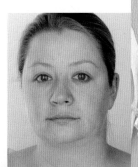

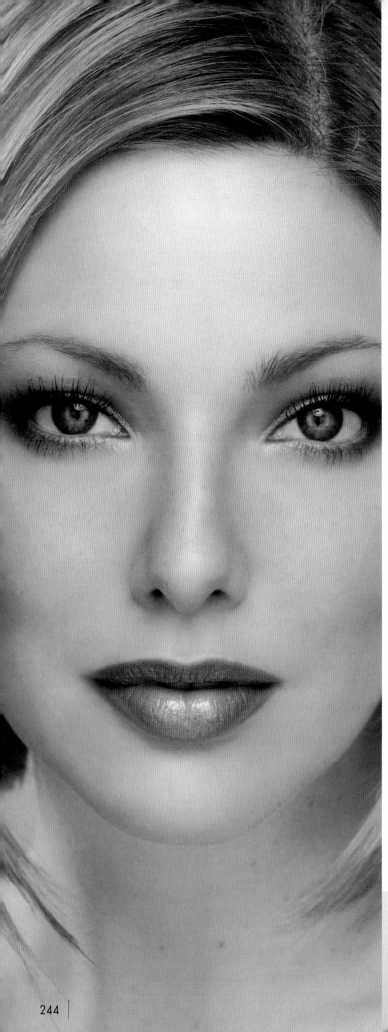

kate

WEDDING TIME:	morning/midday/ late afternoon/evening
EYESHADOW APPLICATION:	sparkling eye (page 222)
EYESHADOW:	highlight: matte nude/ shimmer flesh midtone: matte taupe contour: matte mahogany
BLUSH:	rich honey
LIP LINER:	deep coral
LIPSTICK:	warm pink
LIP GLOSS:	shimmer coral
TIPS:	To make the shimmer highlight eyeshadow shade show the most, I first layered a matte nude color on the lid (to create a base), then applied the shimmer highlight eyeshadow shade on top to make it stand out even more. I chose not to use any eyeliner, and instead got all my lash definition from using contour eyeshadow shade all along the lashline along with lots of thick dark lashes. This is such a great look because it works at any time of day!

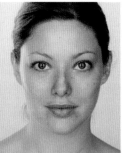

nonna

WEDDING TIME:	morning/midday/late afternoon
EYESHADOW APPLICATION:	sparkling eye (page 222)
EYESHADOW:	highlight: shimmer gold midtone: matte caramel blush: rich honey
LIP LINER:	flesh
LIPSTICK:	pinkish nude
LIP GLOSS:	creamy nude
TIPS:	I wanted a soft monochromatic look, so I used varying degrees of the same colors. To make the eyes even more subtle, I only used a highlight and midtone, and didn't use any eyeliner. In order to get more eye definition, I simply defined the lashline with the midtone eyeshadow shade and thick dark lashes. To continue the subtle monochromatic look, I used subtle cheek and lip color in the same shade family. Overall, this treatment gives you a soft, natural, glowing look!

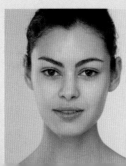

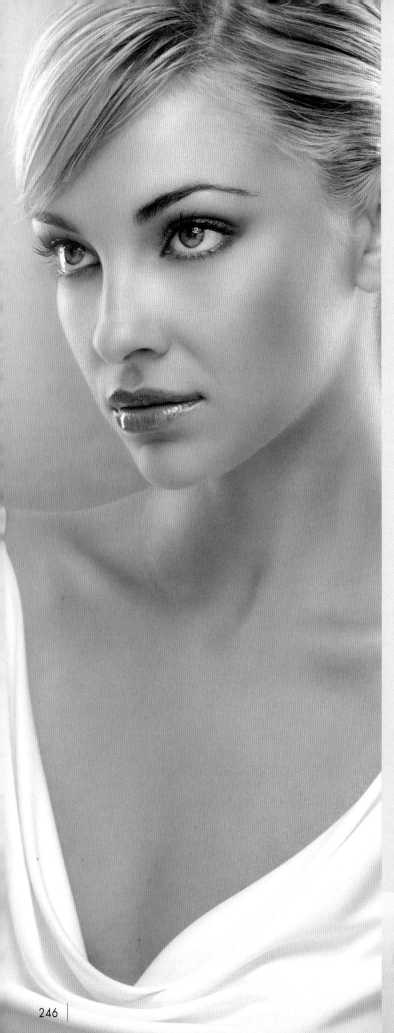

glenna

WEDDING TIME:	morning/midday/ late afternoon/evening
EYESHADOW APPLICATION:	natural beauty (page 217)
EYESHADOW:	highlight: shimmer flesh midtone: matte taupe contour: shimmer golden brown
EYELINER:	bronze
BLUSH:	soft peach
LIP LINER:	flesh
LIPSTICK:	pinkish nude
LIP GLOSS:	shimmer coral
TIPS:	You can never go wrong with subtle beauty when it comes to a bride. For Glenna, I chose soft, warm, natural shades from eyes to lips. I have created definition without overpowering her own true beauty!

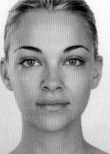

fabiana

WEDDING TIME:	late afternoon/evening
EYESHADOW APPLICATION:	natural beauty (page 217)
EYESHADOW:	highlight: shimmer flesh midtone: matte taupe contour: shimmer golden brown
EYELINER:	rich brown
BLUSH:	rich honey
LIP LINER:	fleshy pink
LIPSTICK:	warm pink
LIP GLOSS:	shimmer berry
TIPS:	Because I have chosen a bit richer lip color, it pushes this look to late afternoon and evening. If I lightened the lip color up a bit and used a little less eyeshadow contour color, this look could work at any time of day. But of course I wanted drama!

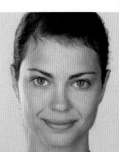

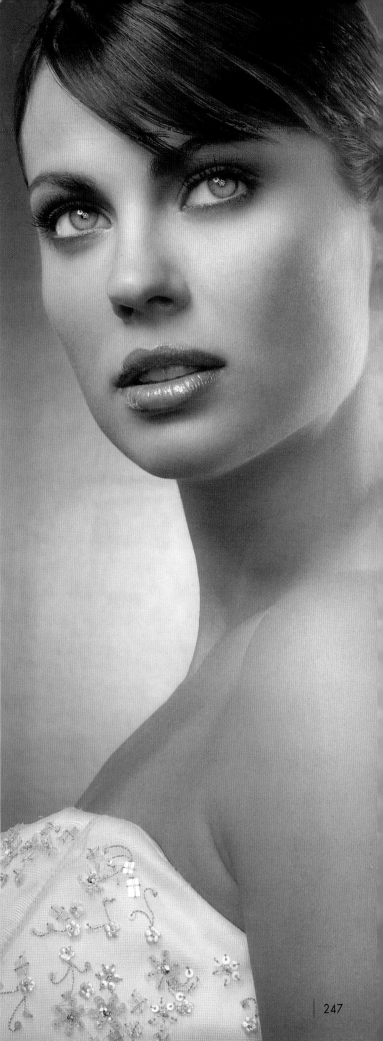

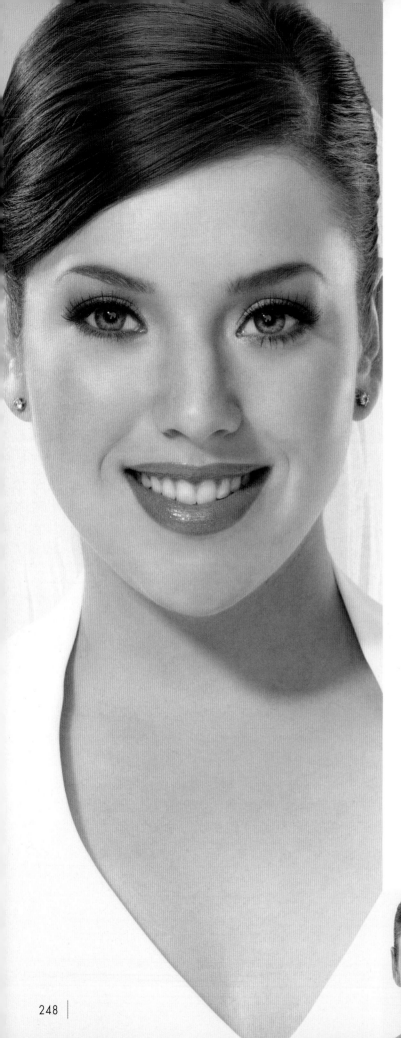

joy

WEDDING TIME:	midday/late afternoon/evening
EYESHADOW APPLICATION:	natural beauty (page 217)
EYESHADOW:	highlight: shimmer gold midtone: matte taupe contour: shimmer chocolate
EYELINER:	bronze
BLUSH:	soft peach
LIP LINER:	deep coral
LIPSTICK:	soft peach
LIP GLOSS:	shimmer coral
TIPS:	For Joy I went for total glamour. Joy is our resident sweet, adorable diva, and I wanted to make sure she was the center of the universe on her special day. I chose very natural shades, and applied them with a bit more intensity for a little more drama. This look would be perfect for any bride, but more importantly, it is the perfect look for "Princess Joy!"

susan

WEDDING TIME:	morning/midday/ late afternoon/evening
EYESHADOW APPLICATION:	natural beauty (page 217)
EYESHADOW:	highlight: shimmer flesh midtone: matte taupe contour: shimmer golden brown
EYELINER:	bronze
BLUSH:	warm pink
LIP LINER:	warm caramel
LIPSTICK:	soft peach
LIP GLOSS:	shimmer warm pink
TIPS:	Choosing subtle, natural shades will always make a look work at any time of day. Here, I made sure to (as always) bronze first, then I chose a blush that would give Susan's face a soft, flushed glow. Pretty skin always makes a pretty picture!

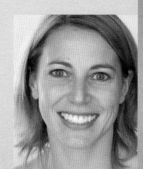

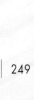

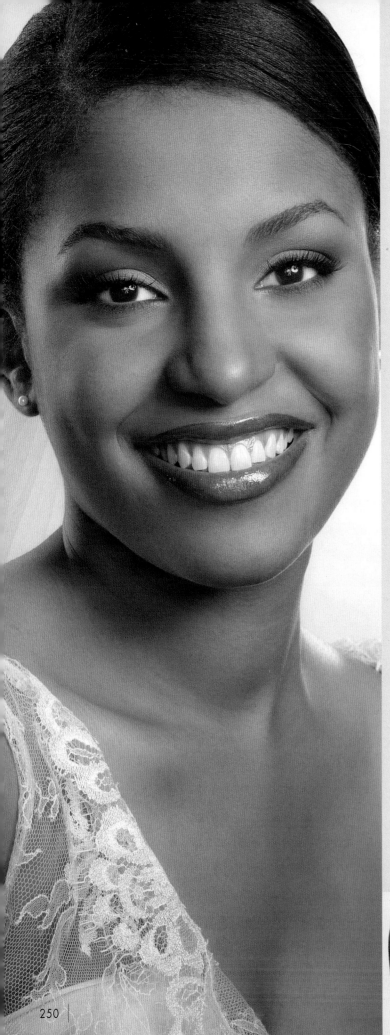

kim

WEDDING TIME:	late afternoon/evening
EYESHADOW APPLICATION:	natural beauty (page 217)
EYESHADOW:	highlight: matte sand midtone: matte mahogany contour: matte charcoal
EYELINER:	charcoal
BLUSH:	rich terracotta
LIP LINER:	warm caramel
LIPSTICK:	golden nude
LIP GLOSS:	shimmer berry
TIPS:	I went a bit more dramatic for Kim's look. I chose a very intense eyeshadow contour color so that the attention would be on her eyes. Of course, with eyes that are a bit more dramatic like this, I made sure that her lip color was very subtle, choosing to get all the color from the gloss and not the lipstick.

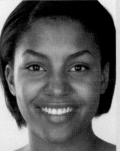

tiffany

WEDDING TIME:	morning/midday/ late afternoon/evening
EYESHADOW APPLICATION:	natural beauty (page 217)
EYESHADOW:	highlight: shimmer flesh midtone: matte dark taupe contour: shimmer chocolate
EYELINER:	rich brown
BLUSH:	rich honey
LIP LINER:	flesh
LIPSTICK:	soft peach
LIP GLOSS:	shimmer warm pink
TIPS:	Talk about a princess! Tiffany could get married at any time of day with her look. (It is never wrong to wear a tiara!) I really gave her skin a lot of color and glow with bronzer. By adding a bit of color and depth to the skin, I made sure it will photograph beautifully, even in the evening with a flash.

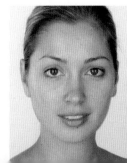

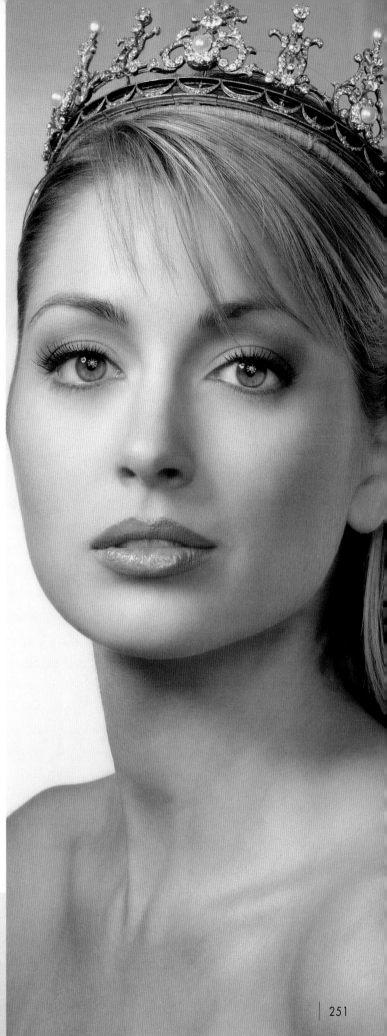

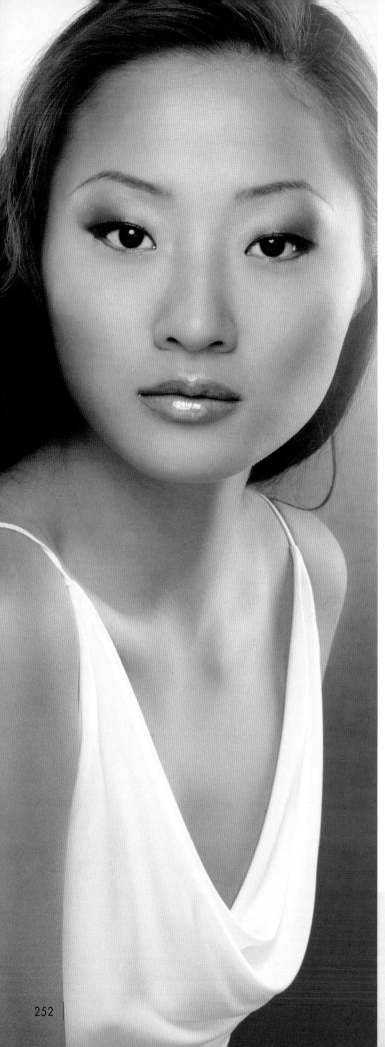

sylvia

WEDDING TIME:	late afternoon/evening
EYESHADOW APPLICATION:	natural beauty (page 217)
EYESHADOW:	highlight: shimmer beige midtone: matte taupe contour: matte dark brown
EYELINER:	rich brown
BLUSH:	rich honey
LIP LINER:	flesh
LIPSTICK:	pinkish nude
LIP GLOSS:	shimmer coral
TIPS:	Normally, a look like Sylvia's would have also worked for midday, but I chose to apply a contour eyeshadow shade with more intensity, so this look works better in the late afternoon or evening. Also, since I intensified the eyes, I kept the cheeks and lips subtle.

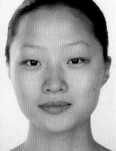

alyssa

WEDDING TIME:	morning/midday/ late afternoon/evening
EYESHADOW APPLICATION:	natural beauty (page 217)
EYESHADOW:	highlight: shimmer flesh midtone: matte taupe contour: shimmer golden brown
EYELINER:	bronze
BLUSH:	soft apricot
LIP LINER:	warm caramel
LIPSTICK:	warm pink
LIP GLOSS:	shimmer coral
TIPS:	Alyssa's look works at any time of day because of its soft, subtle application and shade choices. Sometimes it is just as beautiful *not* to draw attention to any one feature on the face. Instead, choose shades that will give the same amount of soft, subtle definition to all your features.

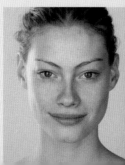

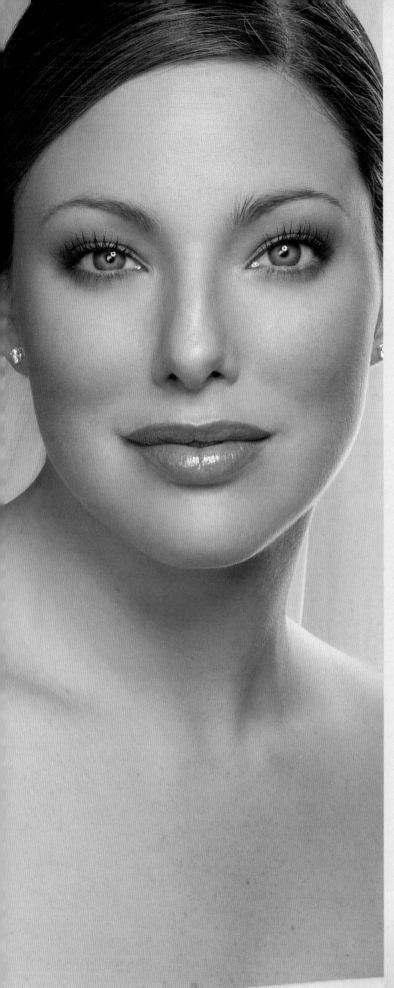

kate

WEDDING TIME:	morning/midday/ late afternoon/evening
EYESHADOW APPLICATION:	natural beauty (page 217)
EYESHADOW:	highlight: shimmer flesh midtone: matte taupe contour: shimmer golden brown
BLUSH:	rich honey
LIP LINER:	flesh
LIPSTICK:	pinkish nude
LIP GLOSS:	shimmer coral
TIPS:	What can I say, other than this is the perfect balance of beauty and definition? I've brought out every feature, without one feature overpowering another. I also chose not to use eyeliner. Instead, I simply used my contour eyeshadow shade to define Kate's eyes all along the lashline. And don't forget thick, gorgeous lashes!

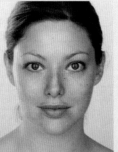

poppi

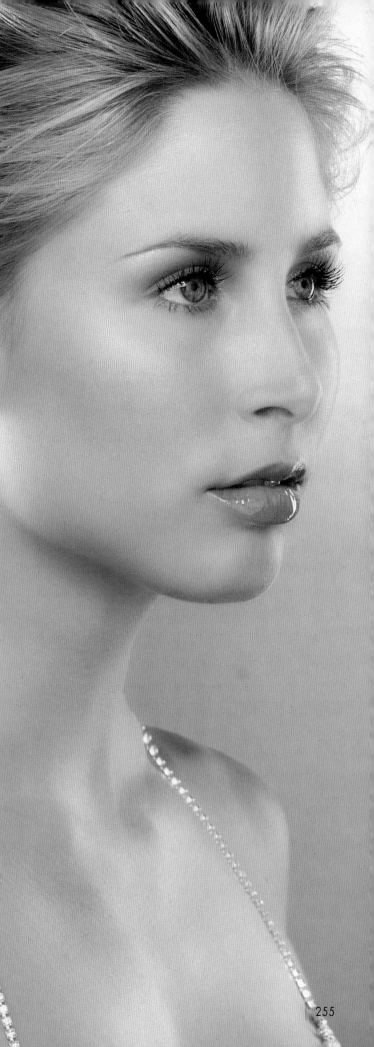

WEDDING TIME:	morning/midday/late afternoon
EYESHADOW APPLICATION:	sparkling eye (page 222)
EYESHADOW:	highlight: matte nude/ shimmer beige midtone: matte rose contour: matte dark taupe
BLUSH:	warm pink
LIP LINER:	flesh
LIPSTICK:	warm pink
LIP GLOSS:	creamy nude
TIPS:	To make the shimmer highlight eyeshadow shade show the most, I first layered a matte nude color on the lid (to create a base), then applied the shimmer highlight eyeshadow shade on top to make it stand out even more. To keep this look the ultimate in natural, I chose not to use any eyeliner. I simply defined the lashline with the contour eyeshadow shade and thick, dark lashes.

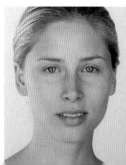

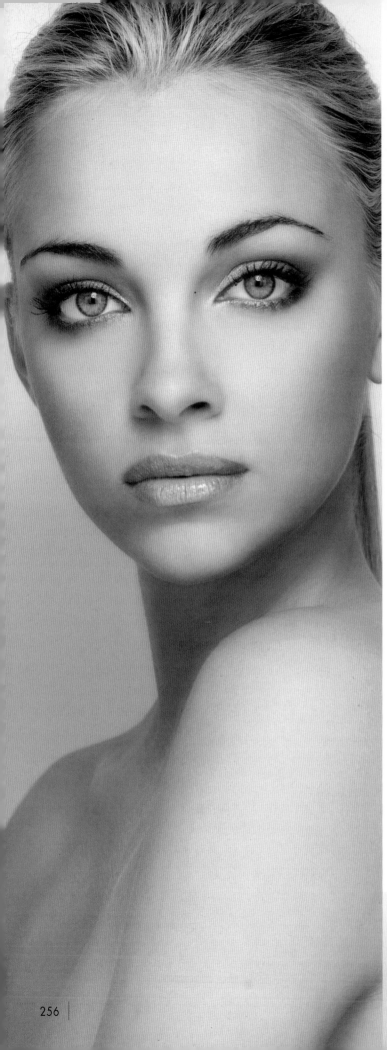

glenna

WEDDING TIME:	late afternoon/evening
EYESHADOW APPLICATION:	natural beauty (page 217)
EYESHADOW:	highlight: shimmer flesh midtone: matte taupe contour: shimmer purple
EYELINER:	purple
BLUSH:	soft peach
LIP LINER:	flesh
LIPSTICK:	pinkish nude
LIP GLOSS:	creamy nude
TIPS:	Okay, I couldn't stand it any longer! I needed a little fun and color. However, adding some color to Glenna's palette limits what times of day her look is appropriate. This look is definitely for a bride who is a glamour girl and wants to play with color.

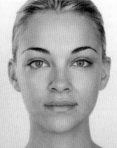

cynthia

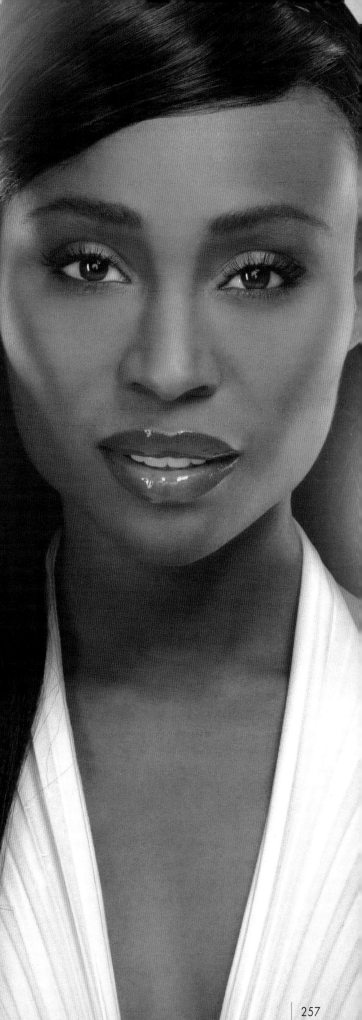

WEDDING TIME:	late afternoon/evening
EYESHADOW APPLICATION:	natural beauty (page 217)
EYESHADOW:	highlight: shimmer gold midtone: matte mahogany contour: shimmer purple
EYELINER:	charcoal
BLUSH:	rich terracotta
LIP LINER:	warm caramel
LIPSTICK:	golden nude
LIP GLOSS:	creamy nude
TIPS:	Drama, drama, drama—sometimes it is the only way to go! This is a look Cynthia can definitely pull off. I just want to remind you that whenever you're creating a dramatic eye look, you always want to keep the lips soft and natural. And it never hurts to make them glossy and shiny. You know every man wants to kiss those lips!

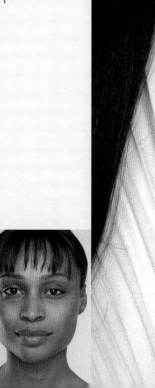

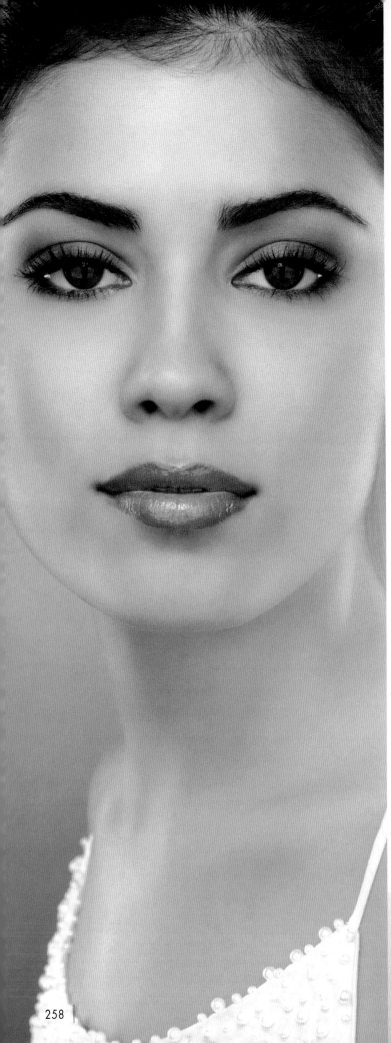

lauren

WEDDING TIME:	evening
EYESHADOW APPLICATION:	smoky eye (page 221)
EYESHADOW:	highlight: shimmer flesh midtone: matte taupe contour: shimmer purple
EYELINER:	purple
BLUSH:	soft apricot
LIP LINER:	flesh
LIPSTICK:	soft peach
LIP GLOSS:	shimmer coral
TIPS:	The bride is supposed to be the center of attention, and Lauren definitely will be! This is a very strong look that I would only do for an evening wedding. I probably would also not choose this look for a blonde, but because of Lauren's coloring, she wears it well.

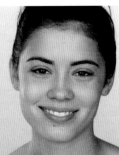

nonna

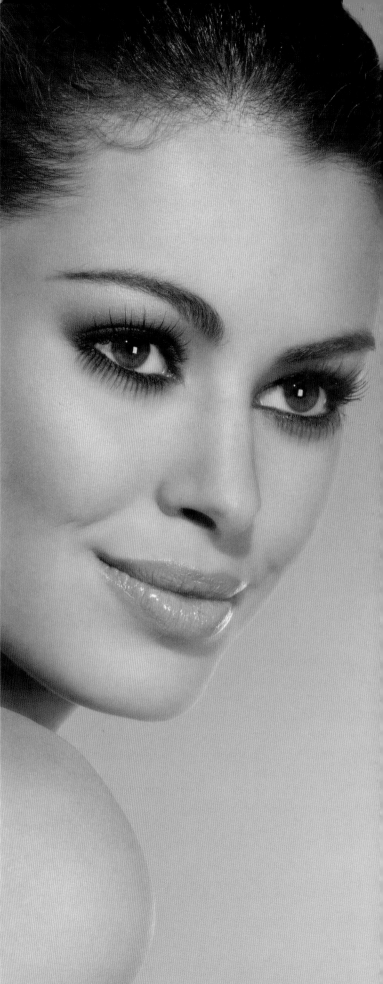

WEDDING TIME:	evening
EYESHADOW APPLICATION:	smoky eye (page 221)
EYESHADOW:	highlight: shimmer gold midtone: matte taupe contour: matte charcoal
EYELINER:	charcoal
BLUSH:	warm pink
LIP LINER:	flesh
LIPSTICK:	pinkish nude
LIP GLOSS:	shimmer coral
TIPS:	Nonna's look is the perfect example of a smoky bridal eye. I used simple, natural shades to make it as subtle a look as a smoky eye can be. You get great drama without it being too much. This look is only for the evening bride. Don't forget to choose a soft, natural nude lip for the perfect balance.

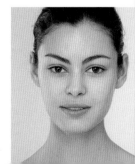

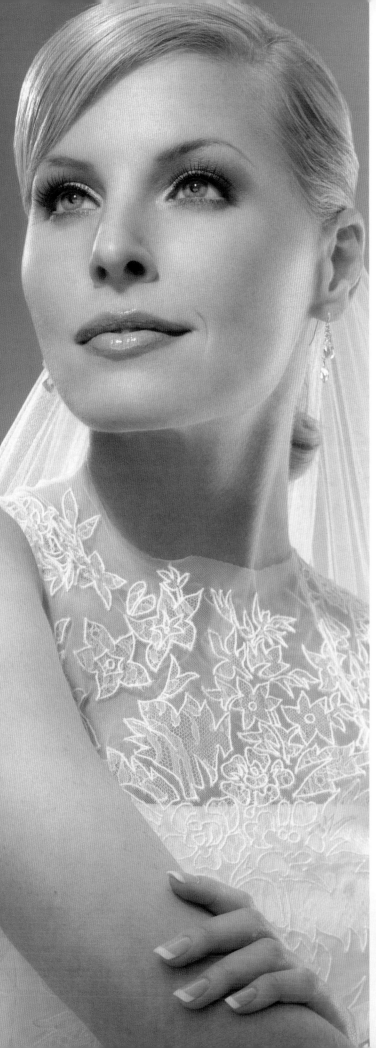

kiley

WEDDING TIME:	late afternoon/evening
EYESHADOW APPLICATION:	sparkling eye (page 222)
EYESHADOW:	highlight: matte nude/ shimmer beige midtone: matte taupe contour: matte mahogany
EYELINER:	rich brown
BLUSH:	warm pink
LIP LINER:	flesh
LIPSTICK:	soft peach
LIP GLOSS:	shimmer coral
TIPS:	To make the shimmer highlight eyeshadow shade show the most, I first layered a matte nude color on the lid (to create a base), then applied the shimmer highlight eyeshadow shade on top to make it stand out even more. I still defined really well at the lashline with liner and thick, dark lashes. Normally, this is a look that works well at midday, but since I chose a bit darker contour eyeshadow shade and a dark liner, it is better for late afternoon or evening.

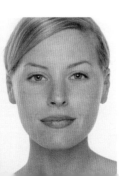

eleanor

WEDDING TIME:	evening
EYESHADOW APPLICATION:	smoky eye (page 221)
EYESHADOW:	highlight: shimmer flesh midtone: matte dark taupe contour: matte mahogany
EYELINER:	rich brown
BLUSH:	rich honey
LIP LINER:	warm caramel
LIPSTICK:	soft peach
LIP GLOSS:	shimmer berry
TIPS:	Glamour was the goal of the day, and I achieved it. I chose a smoky eye with rich, subtle color to create a look that everyone will notice. By not choosing eyeshadow shades that are too dark, we get the drama without it being overpowering. I needed a subtle lip look because of the dramatic eyes, but I wanted a touch of color, so I used a soft natural lipstick, then layered a sheer berry gloss with shimmer on top. This gives the lips a little more depth and color without being too much.

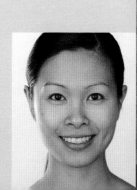

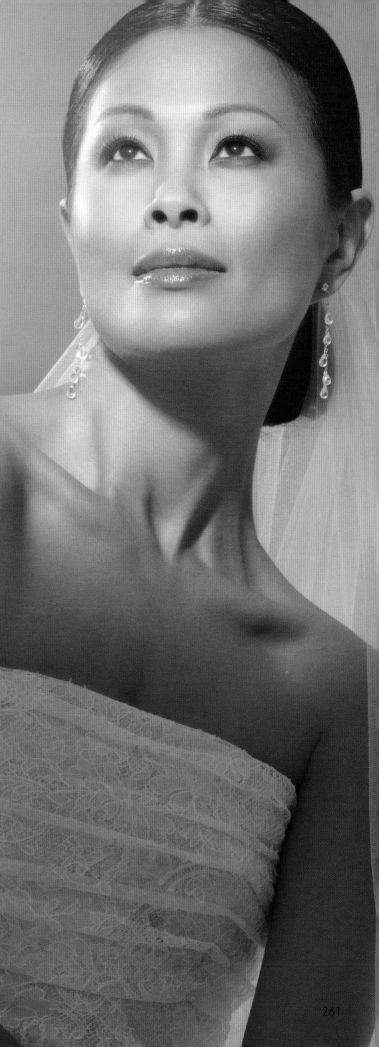

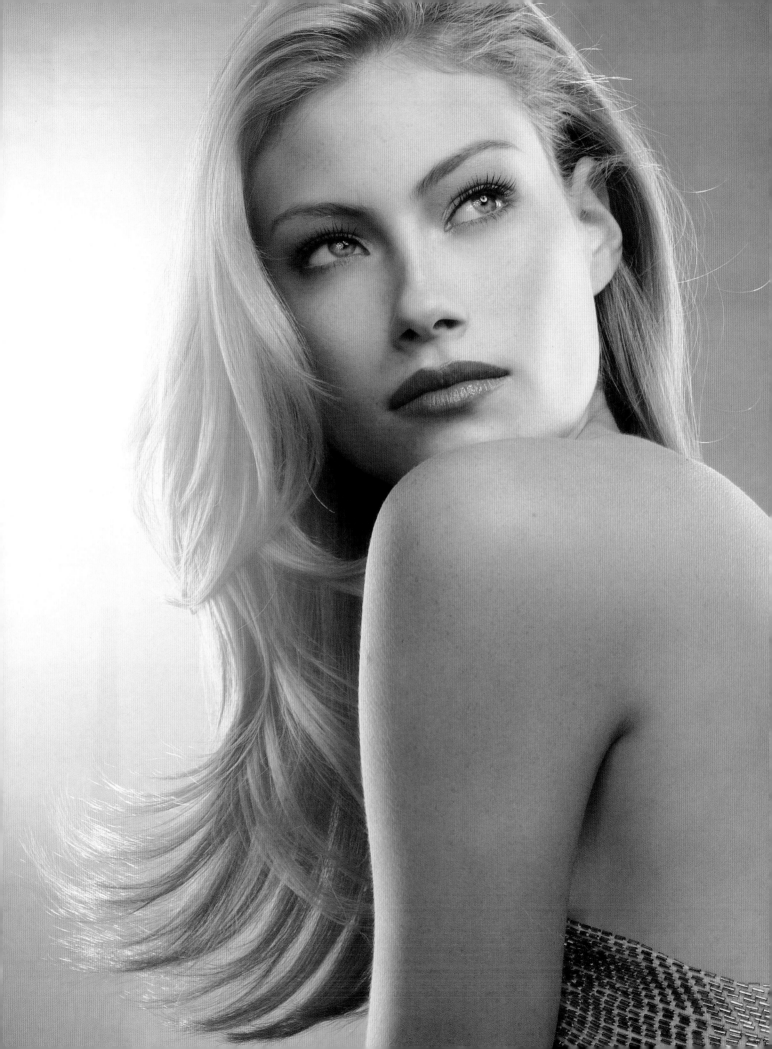

bridesmaids

There are many myths when it comes to makeup looks for bridesmaids. For many years, bridesmaids have been forced to all wear the same makeup colors and shades, no matter what their skin tone. I have looked at so many wedding photos and felt so sorry for all those bridesmaids! First, so often they are made to wear a dress that they never would have picked out for themselves. Then they are forced to wear makeup that is not flattering on top of it. No wonder so many of them end up feeling so unattractive. What a day!

Brides, I appeal to you to have pity on your bridesmaids. Think how *you* would feel in their place! Just as I've shown you how to look beautiful on your special day, I'd like for you to share this chapter with your bridesmaids so they can look and feel beautiful, too. You can all have fun together trying your new makeup looks, and just think how much happier everyone will be! Don't worry—I won't let them upstage you, I promise. After all, it is *your* day!

Let's talk about ways to make your bridesmaids feel beautiful, too. First, as with the bride, we do not want anything too bold or bright, since it will never photograph well. Leaning on the more natural side is the safest and best way to assure beautiful pictures. But you always want to let your bridesmaids feel like themselves. Take into consideration who they are and how they normally wear their makeup—that's what makes them feel beautiful. For the most part, they can still do just that—we just might need to adjust it slightly.

I have some facts and some opinions to share with you. Using this basic information can help create beautiful photographs without stripping each bridesmaid of her individuality. Believe it or not, this can really help your special day flow much more smoothly without unneeded drama. We all know that a woman who feels beautiful is a happy woman.

So here are the facts and a few opinions, of course based on much experience and trial and error.

1. **A bridesmaid's makeup does not have to match her dress.** Makeup is meant to make the girl look more beautiful, not the outfit. Always choose shades that will bring out the girl and her features.

2. **Every girl does not have to wear the same shades of makeup.** There are so many skin tones, we have to consider what each one needs. The only thing that has to match is the intensity of color. You do not want one girl with bold eye makeup and one with almost none. I think a subtle yet defined look always looks good and will photograph perfectly.

3. **Every girl does not have to wear the same shade of lipstick.** I know that this is the most common piece of makeup that everyone thinks just has to match. Once again, the same shade will not look perfect on every girl. The only aspect of the color that has to match is the intensity. You do not want one girl in bold or deep lip color and another in a nude lip color. Once again, a subtle shade that defines yet adds color will always photograph flawlessly.

4. **Have the bride and bridesmaids look the opposite of one another.** This is one thing that I have found really sets the bride apart from the bridesmaids. What I mean by this is: If the bride wears her hair up, all the bridesmaids should wear theirs down. If the bride wears her hair down, all the bridesmaids should wear theirs up. I know this might seem trivial, but in my experience, this makes for beautiful photographs and it helps the bride really stand out.

5. **Most importantly, you never want the bridesmaids' makeup to be more intense than the bride's.** You never want the bridemaids' look to overshadow the bride's! It is her special day, and it is all about her. They are there in a supporting role.

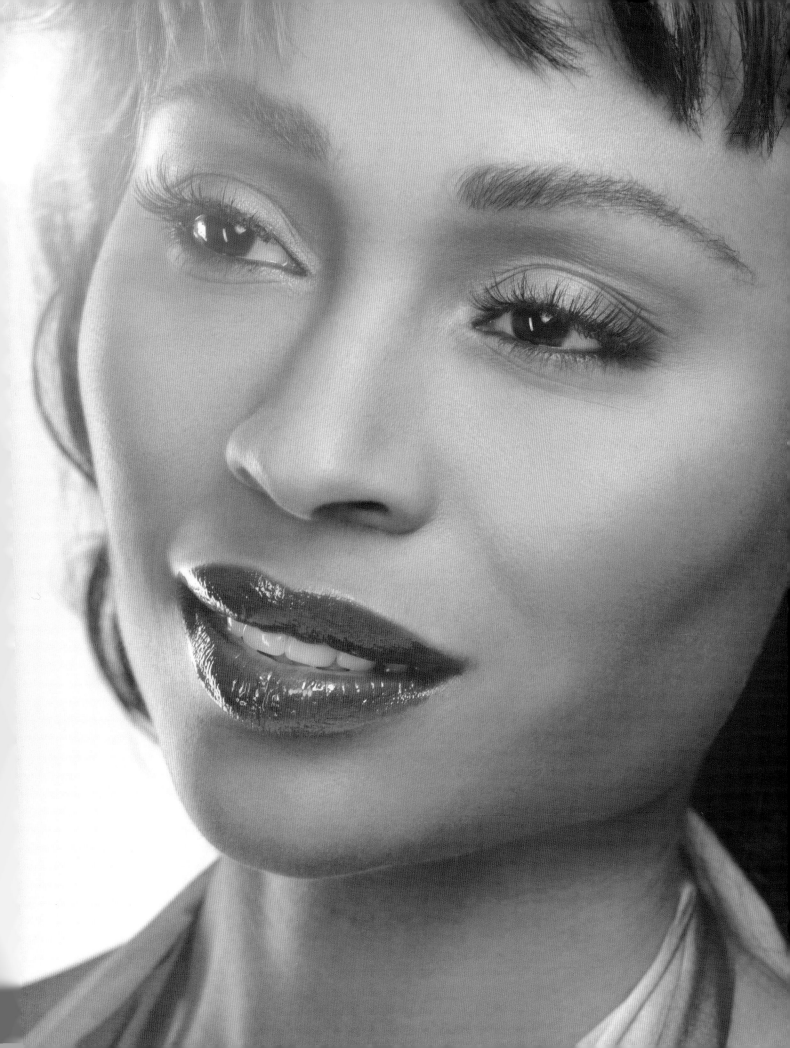

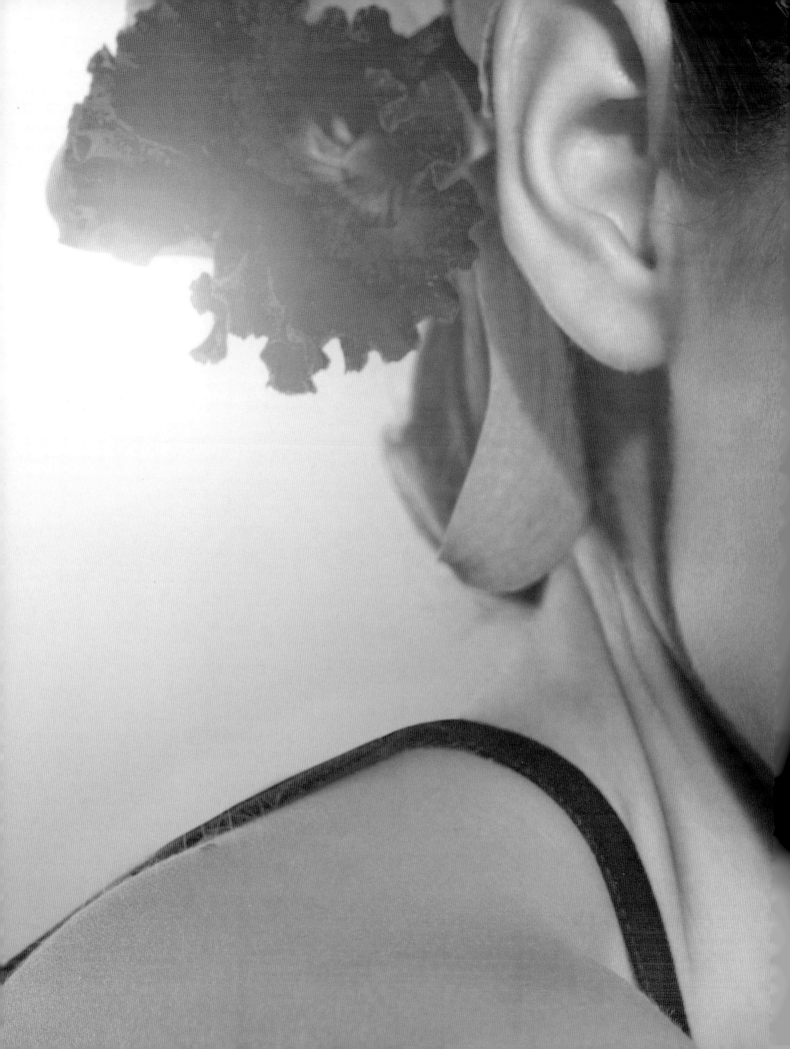

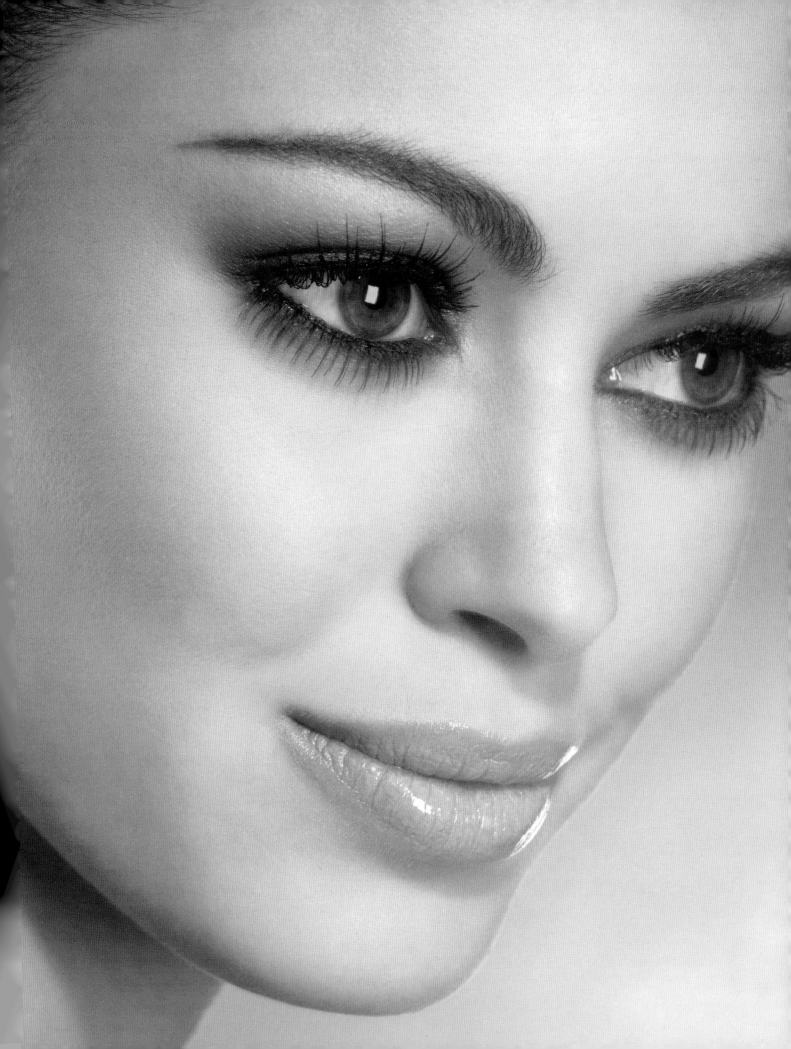

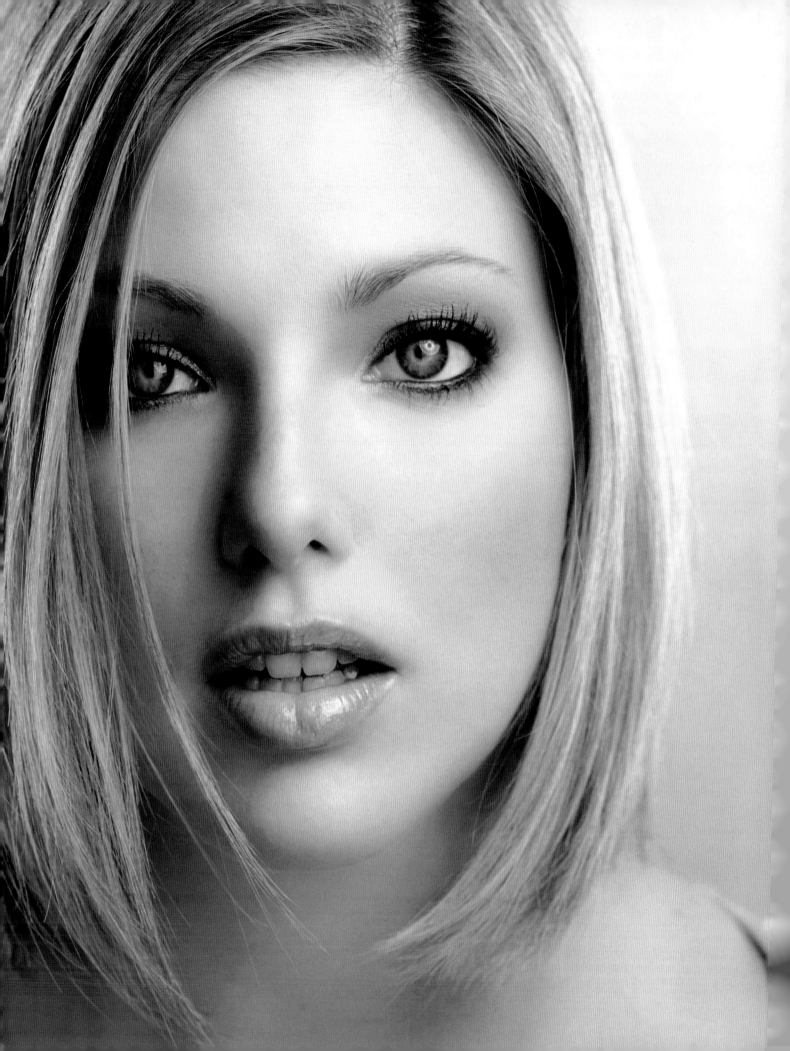

afterword

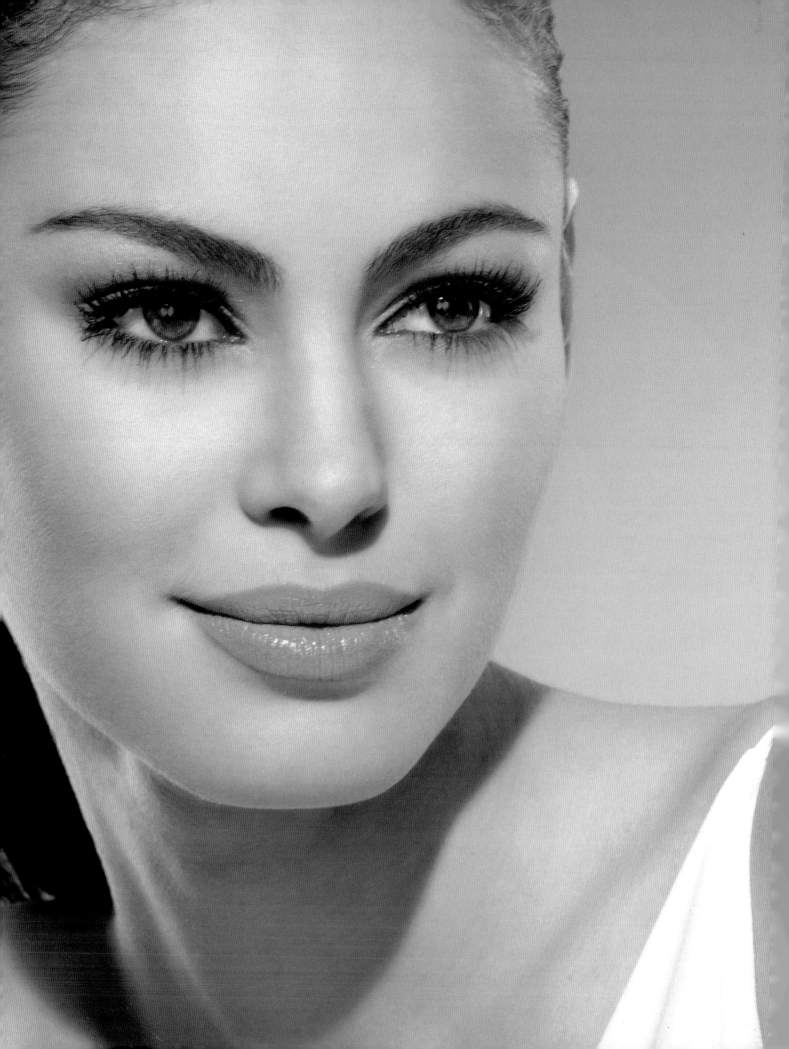

Throughout the years, I have been surrounded by beautiful, strong women, all of whom have greatly influenced my ideals of beauty. My training in beauty began with many years of studying art, which I think is why I pay particular attention to the importance of shading, undertones, and blending. My maternal grandfather was a talented artist and painter, so when my mother noticed very early on that I exhibited a similar gift, I was encouraged to begin studying. As early as the sixth grade, I won a scholarship to study painting and sculpture at the Museum of Fine Arts in Houston.

After many years of studying painting, I grew tired of it, so I decided to focus my energy on acting. I then attended a high school for the performing arts and majored in theatre. That's where my interest in makeup really began, because along with performing in the productions, I was encouraged to do the makeup for them. Actually, it is there that I received my strongest encouragement to pursue my God-given talents in beauty. I then continued my education by studying all aspects of beauty, including hair and skin.

For as long as I can remember, I have always been mesmerized by glamour. Like a lot of people of my generation, from a very early age I considered "Barbie" to be the absolute epitome of beauty and glamour. I have three sisters, and growing up we spent hours playing "Barbie." As far as I was concerned she had it all—beauty and brains.

Growing up, it was just me and five women. Along with my sisters, there was my mom, who was single, and my grandmother, who was devoted to us. They each had their own style and weren't afraid to express it. I remember from a very young age begging my mother to grow her hair long and to wear dresses. I guess you could say I was destined for the fashion and beauty business. I remember going (sometimes once a week) with my mother and grandmother to the beauty shop, watching them get their hair done and loving the experience.

One of my fondest childhood memories is of standing watching my grandmother with vast interest as she applied her makeup. Her eyebrows were always a little too dark and slightly crooked. I remember rosy-pink overdone cheeks and frosted, "cotton-candy" pink lipstick. "Nonna" wore her makeup faithfully every single day. In fact, I never saw her go anywhere without it.

Another fond memory is of my mother as she prepared for a date in the very early '70s. It was becoming the latest thing to use mascara on the bottom lashes, and I remember sitting watching her and her look of concentration as she carefully applied it for the very first time. When she finished she turned to me and announced she felt that she looked a bit like Raggedy Ann. Of course, I thought she looked fabulous.

Then there were my sisters. Occasionally, as we got older, I was able to practice hair and makeup on them. It didn't happen that often when we were young, because my mother thought boys should not play with hair or paint faces. I still remember getting my younger sisters (who are twins) ready for their prom. I started with helping them shop for their dresses and finished by doing their hair and makeup for that special night. I guess I have always loved the transformation process.

Since education and knowledge is strength, I can only hope that the information compiled in my book will encourage you, boost your self-confidence, and help you to reveal your true beauty.

As we end our time together, I want to leave you with this thought: Beauty isn't just about makeup. It's about self-confidence, individuality, and the desire to embrace your inner beauty. These are the beauty marks that really make you unforgettable. Wear them proudly every day, along with a smile and your own sense of style, and you'll be absolutely beautiful, inside and out.

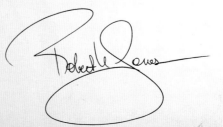

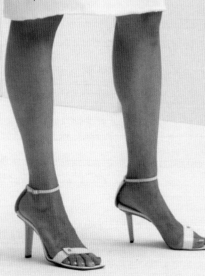

self-confidence is the most important element of true beauty.

—robert jones